Manual of Acute Pain Management in Children

Edited by

Ian M. McKenzie

Anaesthetist, Royal Children's Hospital, Melbourne

Phillip B. Gaukroger

Paediatric Anaesthetist, Women's and Children's Hospital, Adelaide

Philip G. Ragg

Anaesthetist, Royal Children's Hospital, Melbourne

T.C.K. (Kester) Brown

Director of Anesthesia, Royal Children's Hospital, Melbourne

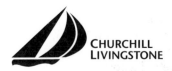

CHURCHILL
LIVINGSTONE

NEW YORK EDINBURGH LONDON MADRID MELBOURNE SAN FRANCISCO AND TOKYO 1997

CHURCHILL LIVINGSTONE
Medical Division of Pearson Professional Limited

Distributed in the United States of America by Churchill Livingstone
Inc., 650 Avenue of the Americas, New York, NY 10011, and by
associated companies, branches and representatives throughout the
world.

© Pearson Professional Limited 1997

First published 1997

ISBN   0-443-05321-9

British Library Cataloguing in Publication Data
A catalogue record for this book is available from the British Library.

Library of Congress Cataloging in Publication Data
A catalog record for this book is available from the Library of Congress.

Medical knowledge is constantly changing. As new information becomes available,
changes in treatment, procedures, equipment and the use of drugs become necessary. The
editors/authors/contributors and the publishers have, as far as it is possible, taken care that
the information given in this text is accurate and up to date. However, readers are strongly
advised to confirm that the information, especially with regard to drug usage, complies
with the latest legislation and standards of practice.

Produced by Longman Asia Ltd, Hong Kong
SWT/01

Manual of Acute Pain Management in Children

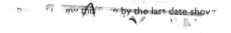
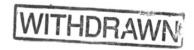
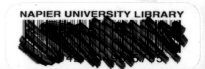

The editors would like to acknowledge the help of the Educational Resources Centre of the Royal Children's Hospital, particularly Mr Bill Reid, in the preparation of the drawings and figures in this volume.

For Churchill Livingstone:
Commissioning Editor: Gavin Smith
Project Controller: Sarah Lowe
Cover Design: Jeannette Jacobs
Copy Editor: Anne Ashford
Indexer: John Sampson

Contents

Contributors

Jag Ahluwalia BA BChir MB BA DRCOG DCH MRCGP MRCP (UK)
Fellow in Neonatology, Royal Children's Hospital, Melbourne

Roger Allen MB BS FRACP
Paediatrician, Rheumatologist, Royal Children's Hospital, Melbourne

Peter Barnett MB BS MSc FRACP FACEM
Deputy Director, Department of Emergency Medicine, Royal Children's
Hospital, Melbourne

Katrina E Brereton MRN RN ND
Clinical Nurse Co-ordinator – Acute Pain Management Service, Royal
Children's Hospital, Melbourne

T CK (Kester) Brown MD FANZCA FRCA
Director of Anaesthesia, Royal Children's Hospital, Melbourne

Robert L Eyres MB BS FANZCA
Anaesthetist, Royal Children's Hospital, Melbourne

Meredith J Gabriel MB BS BMedSc (Hons) FANZCA
Paediatric Anaesthetist, Women's & Children's Hospital, Adelaide

Phillip B Gaukroger MB BS FANZCA
Senior Consultant Paediatric Anaesthetist, Women's & Children's
Hospital, Adelaide

Robert D Henning FRCA FFICANZCA
Staff Specialist – Intensive Care Unit, Royal Children's Hospital,
Melbourne

John P Keneally MB BS FANZCA
Deputy Director of Anaesthesia, New Children's Hospital, Westmead,
Sydney

Peter Loughnan MB BS FRACP
Paediatrician – Neonatologist, Royal Children's Hospital, Melbourne

Ian M McKenzie MB BS FANZCA
Anaesthetist, Royal Children's Hospital, Melbourne

Philip G Ragg MB BS FANZCA
Anaesthetist, Royal Children's Hospital, Melbourne

Suellen M Walker MB BS FANZCA
Anaesthetist, Royal Children's Hospital, Melbourne

Foreword

It is only in the last two decades that there have been systematic attempts to provide adequate management of pain in children. Before this, little attention was paid to the management of severe acute pain in children. Misconceptions, such as the ideas that it was too dangerous to use many anesthetic and analgesic agents in small children and that young infants did not feel pain or would not be harmed by it, were widely accepted. Since that time, there have been steady improvements in pediatric analgesia. Techniques for pain control in children have been developed through clinical experience, controlled trials and modification of techniques used for adults.

This book has been written by clinicians from a variety of disciplines who manage acute pain in three pediatric hospitals in Australia. These centers have a long history of interest in pediatric pain management. The authors have provided practical accounts of techniques for managing children's pain in different circumstances. The clinical advice and many of the techniques described are appropriate for pain control in children in a wide range of hospitals.

The content and layout of the chapters have been designed to provide ready reference to summaries of clinical aspects of pediatric acute pain management for ward medical, nursing and paramedical staff. Senior staff wishing to improve pain management for children will find discussion of the organizational and educational requirements, as well as protocols for applying modern analgesic techniques. The down-to-earth advice contained in this book will be valuable for all those who manage children with acute pain.

Frank Shann MD, FRACP
Professor of Critical Care Medicine
Royal Children's Hospital, Melbourne

Preface

Intramuscular analgesics given intermittently formed the basis of management of severe pain for many years. As basic pharmacological principles became more widely understood the use of infusions and then patient controlled techniques were introduced. More recent developments in the understanding of pain responses and pharmacology in infants have led to great interest in pain relief in infants and children in recent years. Local anesthetic nerve blocks and regional techniques have increasingly been used in infants and children and now epidurals with local and other analgesic drugs are quite commonly used in many pediatric centers.

This manual has been written by staff – anesthetists, physicians and a nurse – of the Children's Hospitals in Melbourne, Adelaide and Sydney. Each has contributed in areas of their special expertise but each chapter has been reviewed by three or four others to ensure that a broad view of each subject is presented.

The aim has been to provide a concise, easy to read, practical and informative manual for use by anyone involved in acute pain management who wants to know the basic information and how to provide analgesia for infants and children. It does not aim to be a reference text as several of these are already available.

TCK (Kester) Brown

Drug terminology

The American names for drugs have been used throughout the book. The following are their English equivalents:

acetaminophen = paracetamol

meperidine = pethidine

epinephrine = adrenaline

lidocaine = lignocaine

tetracaine = amethocaine

succinylcholine = suxamethonium

1 Introduction

Ian McKenzie

The management of acute pain in children was until recently a neglected area of medical and nursing practice. In 1976, a major center published the results of patent ductus arteriosus ligation in premature infants describing an 'anesthesia' technique using oxygen and the muscle relaxant pancuronium. No anesthesia or analgesia was used for these thoracotomies. Today, this protocol would not be approved by an animal ethics committee, let alone be acceptable in the management of children. In the 1980s, a number of studies demonstrated very limited use of analgesics in children even after major surgery. The following 10 years have seen a huge increase in interest in pediatric analgesia. Developments in pain assessment (a particular problem in younger children), monitoring (Ch. 11), analgesic techniques suitable for children (often modified from adult practice), and acute pain management services (Ch. 23) now make provision of good pain relief a routine goal in pediatric practice.

Most pain experienced by children in hospital is acute. A common reason for inadequate relief of acute pain in children is inadequate education of staff (Ch. 12). Good pain management is possible without sophisticated devices such as syringe drivers, patient-controlled analgesia (PCA), or epidural infusions. The information explosion in pediatric pain has produced an extensive academic literature and excellent major texts covering the whole spectrum of pain management.[1] The aim of this book is to provide all staff involved with a summary of the basic science, rationale, and practical management of acute pain in children.

WHY HAS PAIN RELIEF BEEN SO LONG COMING TO CHILDREN?

Children usually heal rapidly, recovery from major surgery often taking only a few days. Even if their pain is not well managed they are likely to survive and go home. Poor analgesia will not show up in standard audits of morbidity and mortality. Individual medical and nursing staff may feel that they have done their job if the presenting problem has been treated. It was often accepted that the patient's pain was an inevitable part of their illness and treatment.

Historically, there has been little training in acute pain management and commonly no particular staff member was responsible for treating the patient's pain. This was compounded in pediatrics by unreasonable fear of the complications of analgesics, born of inexperience ('We've never done that'); the fact that most patients recovered anyway; beliefs that small children either did not feel pain or would forget it; the patient's fear of intramuscular injections; and a failure to appreciate the major adverse effects of inadequate pain relief. Respiratory complications or increased catabolic states preventable by adequate pain relief, if noticed, would usually be classified as complications of surgery. Psychological stress, loss of confidence in hospital staff, and fear of future interventions as a consequence of poor pain management were often accepted as inevitable, and were unlikely to be documented. The benefits of good pain management go beyond the simple but humanitarian concept that relieving pain is good in itself. The child is unlikely to be a good advocate for change, and often the child's family may not have the knowledge or confidence to press for better analgesia.

HOW DOES PAIN MANAGEMENT IN CHILDREN DIFFER FROM ADULT PAIN MANAGEMENT?

The differences in pain management between children and adults are dominated by the psychological development of the child (Ch. 2). Assessment (Ch. 10) is confounded by the limited and nonspecific communication (e.g. crying) of small children. The appropriate methods of reassurance and children's understanding of their condition will be determined by their developmental stage. Pharmacodynamic and kinetic differences are of consequence mainly in the neonatal and infant period. The risk of respiratory depression due to opioids is usually similar in adults and normal children aged more than 3 months. Careful titration of reduced doses and increased monitoring and staffing can make opioid use safe in younger and higher-risk patients. A good understanding of the basic pharmacology of analgesic drugs, including indications, contraindications, dosage, and routes of delivery, is essential for the optimal use of these drugs in children. These aspects are covered in Chapters 3–5 for systemic analgesia, and Chapters 7–9 for local anesthesia.

Two examples of the effect of developmental stage on the appropriateness of specific analgesic techniques are provided by intramuscular injections and patient-controlled analgesia (Ch. 6). Children are particularly susceptible to the 'negative conditioning' that painful delivery of analgesia, such as intramuscular injections, may cause. They may choose to tolerate severe pain rather than have an injection. To successfully use PCA children must understand the system. Some as young as 4 years old may be able to do this, but 7 years is the usual minimum age. In younger children similar flexibility can be achieved by training the nursing staff to adjust the rate of opioid infusions and give boluses to match the patient's requirements.

PSYCHOLOGICAL ASPECTS OF ACUTE PAIN MANAGEMENT

The distress, despair, and anger that are experienced by children in pain and their families are exaggerated if they believe that no-one cares. Active pain management with routine pain assessment and a clear plan if inadequate analgesia occurs prevent these reactions, reassuring the patient, the family, and the staff. The plan should include alternative and supplementary analgesia and ready availability of consultation and further assessment. Specific pain management techniques may be more acceptable to the patient and family if the reasons for using the techniques are explained and they know that the treatment is open to review.

The experience of acute pain is greatly affected by the patient's psyche, developmental stage, and the circumstances of the pain stimulus, making psychological management an integral part of acute pain management. Sensitive handling of the child and family and specific techniques, such as distraction during procedures or 'guided imagery', may contribute greatly to pain management. These techniques are discussed in Chapter 13. While good psychological management of a child with acute pain can lessen problems with administration and requirements for the delivery of pharmacological analgesia, the positive psychological effects of good pharmacological analgesia should not be underestimated.

The circumstances of the pain stimulus may influence how hospital staff are perceived. The psychological effect of the pain of medical and surgical conditions where pain is a presenting symptom (Ch. 20) differs from that of acute procedural pain and the pain of most elective surgery. Patients presenting with painful conditions tend to perceive staff as a potential source of relief. Pain-free children requiring surgery or potentially painful procedures quite logically tend to assign the cause of their pain to the staff. The prevention of pain in patients who are pain-free prior to a procedure is vital for the maintenance of the child's confidence in staff.

PERIOPERATIVE PAIN RELIEF

The use of drugs such as acetaminophen (paracetamol), local anesthetic agents, and morphine has become the cornerstone of pediatric perioperative analgesia (Ch. 15). The efficacy of acetaminophen and other 'simple' analgesics is often underestimated (Ch. 3). The commonest errors in acetaminophen usage are to omit it, give it too late, or to underdose. Acetaminophen can be given as a 20–30 mg/kg loading dose preoperatively orally (or rectally after induction of anesthesia), then at a dose of 20 mg/kg with a maximum dosage of 100 mg/kg per 24 hours.

Anesthesiologists want their patients to awaken free of pain. Local anesthesia is often the most effective analgesia. An understanding of the effects of intraoperative local anesthetic agents is important for postoperative care. Surgical and nursing staff have frequently received little formal training in the nature and management of regional anesthesia. Chapters 7–9 cover epidural and nerve block analgesia. Opioids (Ch. 5) are still indicated for most major procedures, but complications – particularly nausea and vomiting – make alternatives attractive.

Physical therapies, such as heat, cold, massage, and exercise, have been used for many years, but only recently have these techniques and newer therapies, such as transcutaneous electrical nerve stimulation (TENS) and acupuncture, achieved more formal recognition and a place in acute pain management of children in some centers. These therapies are discussed in Chapter 13.

The prompt and effective management of complications and problems related to pain therapy can relieve distressing symptoms, allow effective analgesia to continue and maintain patient and family confidence in the techniques and staff (Ch. 14).

ACUTE PAIN MANAGEMENT FOR SPECIFIC CONDITIONS AND CIRCUMSTANCES

Patients who have prolonged or recurrent acute pain often benefit from analgesia based on the long-term or repeated application of the principles of acute pain management. Burns, cancer, and arthritis commonly lead to this sort of clinical scenario. Although the principles are similar, the details of management vary greatly and are discussed in Chapters 16, 17, and 21. Similarly, the details of the pain management of neonates and critically ill patients differ from those of other children and are dealt with in Chapters 18 and 19.

Ward procedural pain may be difficult to manage. The availability of staff trained in the use of boluses of opioids, local anesthesia, sedation, inhaled nitrous oxide (Ch. 4) and nonpharmacological techniques can solve most procedural pain problems.

CHRONIC PAIN

Complex regional pain syndrome type 1 (CRPS-1) (Ch. 22), formerly known as reflex sympathetic dystrophy, usually presents as prolonged, severe acute pain. The diagnosis is often missed and consequently the child is inappropriately managed. The benefits of early detection and correct management of this condition, combined with the likelihood that clinicians dealing with acute pediatric pain will be referred these patients, makes an understanding of the recognition and management of CRPS-1 important.

In general, the management of chronic pain requires a different approach, with many contrasts with acute pain management. Chronic pain is unlikely to resolve rapidly. The origins of chronic pain and the response to analgesics (used in acute pain) are different. The effect of chronic pain on daily living, relationships, and the patient's psyche will often create problems that go beyond the need for pain relief alone. Patients must accept that they must make the best of their life while waiting for their pain to improve. Multidisciplinary management with detailed analysis of the origins of the chronic pain, the secondary problems, in combination with analgesic modalities that differ from acute pain interventions, produces the best results. The management of these patients is beyond the scope of this book.

SUMMARY

Even the most caring and empathetic hospital staff cannot effectively manage children's pain unless they have a range of strategies and the personnel, equipment, knowledge, and time available to implement them. Complications of pain control interventions can be minimized by appropriate training, protocols, monitoring, and resuscitation. This book is an attempt to summarize some practical approaches to the management of acute pain in children.

REFERENCE

1. Schecter NL, Berde CB, Yaster M. (eds) 1993 Pain in infants, children, and adolescents. Williams & Wilkins, Baltimore.

2 Developmental physiology and psychology

Ian McKenzie

INTRODUCTION

Pain is a subjective emotional experience. A child's developmental stage influences both that experience and its expression. The problems of tailoring acute pain management to a child's needs is dominated by the child's stage of development.

DEVELOPMENTAL ASPECTS OF PHYSIOLOGY AND PSYCHOLOGY

The rapid maturation of the nervous system that occurs at birth and in the first year of life, particularly the myelination process, has been used as an argument that infants have less pain sensation. Immature, poorly myelinated nerves do transmit action potentials, but more slowly than mature myelinated nerves. Rapid conduction is critical for the coordination of complex body movements and decreasing response time, which is important in larger creatures responsible for their own defense (e.g. an adult). A baby's acute response to a needle-stick (without local anesthesia) is rapid but nonspecific (crying and generalized withdrawal). Theoretically, this cannot be proved to be a painful experience for the child because a baby cannot describe its subjective experience. Semantically, terms such as 'appears distressed' may be more accurate than 'is in pain'. The old saying, 'If it looks, feels and smells like a rose, it is a rose' is pertinent. In the same way that someone without a sense of smell will identify a rose, clinically it seems reasonable to suggest that the baby crying after needle-stick has had a painful experience, even if an accurate subjective report is missing.

More vexed issues arise when the consequences of immature higher cerebral functions in relation to pain are contemplated. If a painful experience is not remembered, does it matter if the pain is not treated? Few adults have clear memories of their life before they were 3 years old. Can this fact justify not treating infant's pain? Babies who have had a number of heel sticks for blood sampling respond differently to preparation for heel stick compared with babies who have not previously had the procedure. Infants who have had bad experiences in an operating theater may become distressed by painless preparations for theater, such as putting on a gown, or by recognizing the place. As parents often comment, 'He knows what's coming'. Although these children have no overt memories of these experiences as adults, they have learnt and shown evidence of at least medium-term memory when they were infants. There is a clinical suggestion that children who have had major (especially if repeated) painful perioperative experiences as infants are more likely to be anxious about a return to the operating room years later. There is no doubt that failure to relieve pain in adults only because they could not communicate (e.g. after generalized brain damage) or remember the experience (e.g. Korsakoff 'psychosis') would be considered inhumane and unacceptable practice. Children need similar consideration.

The difficulties in assessing pain in infants combined with their lack of clear memory for painful experiences seem to lessen the benefits of pain control. This is compounded by the fact that several groups of patients with these problems (e.g. neonates, children with airway problems) may be at greater risk of complications of the treatment of pain. Although the humanitarian factors mentioned above are important, the concept of *primum non nocere* (first do no harm) is also a cornerstone of medical practice. Recent evidence suggests that harm may come from not treating postoperative pain. Decreased postoperative catabolism and improved respiratory function have been shown in babies with effective pain management after major surgery, adding weight to the indications for good pain control. General patient care to minimize pain is indicated in all patients. The risks and benefits of particular treatments of acute pain must be assessed for each patient.

PSYCHOLOGICAL DEVELOPMENTAL STAGES

Dealing with the variability in psychological development of children provides one of the great challenges of patient care in pediatrics. The following is a simple clinical guide to the phases of psychological development in children.

The infant

Up to about 7 months of age, most infants are happy to be comforted by strangers, as long as their basic needs are satisfied. Their expression of distress seems nonspecific, but someone who knows the child or an experienced care-giver may recognize different behaviors as likely to express different needs.

The toddler

Over the subsequent few years most children are wary of strangers, though repeated or prolonged contact can extend the range of 'significant others' well beyond the immediate family of the child. During these years children are sensitive to changes in their normal routine, and tend to cling to a parent or guardian when apprehensive. This presents a problem to the health professional who needs to treat the child immediately with only limited opportunity to become aquainted with the child. Clearly, care should be taken to perform the intervention in the least distressing way. If possible, the involvement of a positive, relaxed, well-informed guardian in the process can minimize distress.

Preschoolers and early primary school children

Once children reach about 4–5 years old, they are usually familiar with surrogate parent figures such as teachers. Children of this age often take pride in their growing independence, and fortunately for staff often have a naive confidence in the good intentions and skills of health professionals. Staff should strive to fulfill these expectations as they make dealing with this group relatively easy. On the other hand, poorly managed, potentially painful interventions such as intravenous blood sampling or injection for investigation or treatment may leave a child feeling brutalized and suspicious of further intervention.

Late primary school children and adolescents

As children grow older they recognize the fallibility of adults, and develop a general knowledge of medical intervention often based on media reports and nightmarish fantasies. They have a growing sense of personal independence and ambitions to be mature and 'adult' in their behavior, yet are acutely aware of their lack of experience and dependence on family support. The adolescent is also subject to rapid physical development, with increasing concerns about body image. It is no surprise therefore, that faced with medical intervention, these children will often be withdrawn, anxious, and fearful. Younger children in this group (8–11 years) commonly present with some bravado obscuring these internal anxieties. Simple, honest explanation of the practicalities of the situation and discussion of their concerns are more useful than general reassurance, no matter how emphatic. These children especially value having control over their environment. Involving them in their own care and the decision-making about their treatment will often allow these children to maintain that sense of control.

THE PAIN PATHWAY

The understanding of the complex physiology of acute pain sensation continues to grow. The following is a summary of the mechanisms involved.

A peripheral painful stimulus provokes an action potential (or series of action potentials) that carry the information via a sensory nerve to the central nervous system. The stimulus may be mechanical, thermal, or chemical energy which produces an action potential in 'pain-sensing' bare nerve endings, particularly in unmyelinated, slow-conducting C fibers, and small, myelinated Aδ fibers. Tissue injury will damage cell membranes releasing precursors (e.g. arachidonic acid) of the chemical mediators of the inflammatory response (e.g. prostaglandins and leukotrienes) which provide a continuing pain stimulus to nerves. The action potentials pass centrally via the peripheral nerve and then the dorsal spinal nerve root, synapsing in the substantia gelatinosa in the dorsal horn of the spinal cord. This synapse is a complex 'junction box' with inhibitory influences from local encephalinergic interneurons, descending serotonergic and adrenergic nerves, and the activity of other spinal neurons. The likely neurotransmitter of the primary afferent spinal pain fiber is substance P. The secondary pain fibers arising from the dorsal horn cross the midline and ascend in the contralateral spinothalamic tract. The faster-conducting Aδ fibers connect to the fast-conducting neospinothalamic (*neo* – new in an evolutionary sense) tract, allowing rapid transmission of 'sharp' pain and rapid reflex responses. The slower C fibers connect to the paleospinothalamic (*paleo* – old) tract, allowing slow conduction of ongoing dull pain with wide central ramifications, producing the common emotional and autonomic responses to pain. In the region of the periaqueductal gray matter, there is initiation of the negative feedback of the descending inhibitory fibers. The pain impulses pass via the thalamus to radiate widely, not only to the specific post-central cortical gyrus sensory mapping region, but also to the limbic and other regions producing emotional and other responses to pain. The interaction between these areas means that not only does pain affect mood and arousal, but that mood and arousal can affect the pain experience.

One area of controversy in pain management is the clinical significance of 'preemptive analgesia', the practice of treating pain before it occurs in order to minimize the impact on central pain processing. Physiological research findings of 'wind-up' of central nervous system pain processing nerves (an increase in sensitivity in relation to stimulation) provide one rationale for this practice. Within this framework the analgesia should come before the stimulus, even in an anesthetized patient, but clinical studies have produced conflicting results. What is clear clinically is the benefit of analgesia effective before arousal after elective surgery under anesthesia. Children are especially vulnerable to the psychological distress and loss of confidence in staff produced by waking in pain. This psychological distress, humanitarian factors, the difficulties in regaining good pain control in recovery, and the relatively smooth arousal of a pain-free child (which tends to minimize both surgical and anesthetic recovery complications) all contribute to a clear clinical conviction that it is worth ensuring that children emerge from anesthesia with good analgesia.

3 Simple analgesics and sedatives

Meredith Gabriel

Simple analgesics are useful in most types of acute pain and some forms of chronic pain in children. They may be the sole analgesic for lesser degrees of pain but can also supplement other analgesia used in more severe pain. When used as a supplement to opioids, the opioid dose may be reduced and weaning from the opioid facilitated.

ACETAMINOPHEN

Acetaminophen (paracetamol) is the most widely used analgesic and antipyretic drug in pediatric practice. The analgesic effects of acetaminophen have been known since 1893 when clinical studies were first conducted by von Mering who was looking for a synthetic substitute for South American cinchona bark. Acetaminophen has become popular because it provides analgesia without the undesirable side-effects of nonsteroidal antiinflammatory drugs (NSAIDs, see below). It has minimal antiinflammatory activity.

Acetaminophen is available in syrups of many flavors, tablets, capsules, drops, chewable tablets, suppositories and soluble forms. The range of formulations available makes acetaminophen acceptable to the majority of children.

Pharmacology

Acetaminophen is 4-acetamidophenol and is a white, odourless, crystalline powder. It is nonionized and lipid-soluble. Protein binding is negligible with therapeutic plasma concentrations but may increase to 20% in overdosage.

Acetaminophen is metabolized mainly by the liver and to a very small extent by the kidney. The major metabolite is the glucuronide which accounts for half of its biotransformation. The sulfate metabolite accounts for a quarter of acetaminophen metabolism. Oxidative metabolism converts acetaminophen to catechol derivatives or cysteine conjugates but is a minor pathway, less than 20% of a dose being transformed this way. A further metabolic pathway, which is minor at normal therapeutic doses, is via a reactive metabolite which is conjugated with glutathione in the mercapturic acid pathway. It is this minor metabolic pathway which is implicated in acetaminophen hepatotoxicity.

Mode of action

Acetaminophen crosses the blood–brain barrier and exerts a central antipyretic effect, blocking the action of prostaglandin synthetase in the region of the anterior hypothalamus. The analgesic effect of the drug is probably due to blockade of impulse generation at the bradykinin-sensitive chemoreceptors that evoke pain in the periphery.

Postoperative analgesia

Acetaminophen has gained widespread use for postoperative analgesia. Suitable procedures include ear, nose and throat surgery, ophthalmology, minor general surgery, dental procedures, plastic surgery, and diagnostic procedures. It is commonly used to supplement local anesthesia blockade, particularly in day surgery patients.

Postoperative pain is best anticipated and pretreated. With acetaminophen, this is achieved by giving an initial loading dose, timed so that analgesia is achieved when it is required. Administering acetaminophen 20–30 mg/kg orally 30 minutes preoperatively or rectally immediately after induction of anesthesia usually achieves this aim. Postoperatively, doses of 20 mg/kg can be given 4-hourly on a regular basis or as required, if this is more appropriate, up to a maximum of 100 mg/kg per day.

Pediatric illnesses

Pain from acute medical illnesses such as ear and throat infections is usually managed with acetaminophen. The pain is generally short-lived and doses of 15–20 mg/kg are effective. Acetaminophen may be useful in the management of childhood migraine and other more minor headaches. Painful exacerbations of chronic medical illnesses such as Crohn's disease, ulcerative colitis and cystic fibrosis may be treated with acetaminophen.

Antipyresis

Much has been written about the use of acetaminophen as an antipyretic. Despite considerable debate and research, no beneficial effects of antipyresis have been demonstrated in pediatrics even in the management of children with febrile convulsions. Fever increases oxygen consumption, carbon dioxide production and cardiac output. In children with limited cardiorespiratory reserve, control of these deleterious effects of fever by acetaminophen's antipyretic effect seems reasonable.

Many febrile children experience pain related to their illness and the decision to administer acetaminophen in these children is based on patient comfort.

Neonates

Although the use of acetaminophen in neonates has not been well studied, theoretically neonates may be less susceptible to hepatotoxicity because they produce lower levels of potentially toxic acetaminophen metabolites. Clinically, hepatotoxicity from acetaminophen in neonates is extremely rare (see Ch. 18).

Adverse reactions and toxicity

Acetaminophen is perhaps the safest analgesic available. Reported side-effects have been few, and in children serious toxicity is uncommon. In adults, hepatotoxicity due to overdose, usually deliberate and self-administered, is the major adverse reaction and can cause death. Children account for less than 20% of all cases of acetaminophen overdosage and hepatotoxicity is uncommon. Pediatric acetaminophen overdosage usually results from dosage or formulation error or accidental ingestion. The low incidence of severe toxicity in children may be related to a greater capacity to metabolize acetaminophen via nontoxic pathways. Acetaminophen hepatotoxicity has not been described in children at doses of less than 150 mg/kg per 24 hours, and death has not been reported from doses of less than 300 mg/kg per 24 hours. In most reported cases of acetaminophen toxicity in children, as well as excess dosage there are usually risk factors such as malnutrition or chronic illness which may deplete glutathione (which protects against toxicity), or prolonged feverish illness which may have affected hepatic function. Toxicity is unlikely with daily doses up to a recommended maximum of 100 mg/kg per 24 hours. If acute overdose occurs, immediate referral for assessment and possible treatment, especially with methionine or N-acetylcysteine, may be lifesaving and prevent liver damage.

NSAIDs

Nonsteroidal antiinflammatory drugs (NSAIDs) are a widely used, structurally diverse class of drugs which have antiinflammatory, antipyretic, analgesic, and antiplatelet actions. In children, these drugs are useful in controlling pain due to chronic inflammatory diseases such as juvenile rheumatoid arthritis (see Ch. 21), as an adjuvant in the management of bone pain due to childhood cancer (see Ch. 17), and also in the treatment of postoperative pain. Like acetaminophen, NSAIDs are not sedative and are associated with a lower incidence of nausea and vomiting than opioids.

Indomethacin, ibuprofen, diclofenac, and naproxen are presented in formulations suitable for pediatric use. Indomethacin, diclofenac, and naproxen are available as suppositories suitable for children, naproxen and ibuprofen as capsules, and naproxen as a syrup.

The use of aspirin (acetylsalicylic acid) in children has been limited since its association with Reye's syndrome was reported. Aspirin still has a role in pediatrics in the management of arthritis (see Ch. 21), and Kawasaki disease, and for its antiplatelet action in children at risk of thromboembolism, such as those with cardiovascular prostheses.

Pharmacology

The NSAIDs act peripherally by inhibiting the enzyme prostaglandin synthetase which converts arachidonic acid to the prostaglandin endoperoxides. These drugs may also have central effects on nociception, but the mechanisms have yet to be elucidated.

Most NSAIDs are metabolized in the liver to inactive metabolites which are excreted in the urine. As many NSAIDs are weakly acidic drugs, they are strongly bound to plasma proteins. Displacement of drugs such as oral hypoglycemic agents and methotrexate can produce significant drug interactions.

Postoperative pain

The NSAIDs are effective in reducing postoperative pain and have an opioid sparing effect when used in conjunction with opioids for postoperative pain. Concern that their antiplatelet effect will lead to bleeding has limited their routine use for perioperative analgesia. They are potentially useful 2–3 days postoperatively in patients still requiring opioids or troubled by the side-effects of opioids. The risk of bleeding at this time is negligible and oral administration is often feasible.

Oncology

The role of NSAIDs is essential in the management of bone pain in pediatric palliative care, (see Ch. 17). They are very good adjuvants to opioid analgesia and reduce the need for dose escalation of opioid drugs. Their antiplatelet effects reduce their suitability for analgesia outside palliative care in these children. The use of NSAIDs with long half-lives such as naproxen allows long dosing intervals and smooth pain control.

Adverse reactions and toxicity

The NSAIDs have a wide range of adverse effects which have limited their use in pediatric practice. Adverse reactions include platelet inactivation, gastric irritation and bleeding, the exacerbation of asthma, and hepatic and renal dysfunction.

In normal hemostasis, prostaglandin endoperoxides and thromboxane A_2 induce rapid and irreversible platelet aggregation. All NSAIDs, except the salicylates, are reversible inhibitors of cyclooxygenase and thus inhibit platelet aggregation only while they remain in the circulation. This effect on platelet function may cause an increased incidence of bleeding intraoperatively and postoperatively. This has been demonstrated when NSAIDs have been used for analgesia for tonsillectomy.

All NSAIDs have the potential to damage gastric mucosa, probably by the systemic inhibition of prostaglandin synthesis, not just by local irritation. This inhibition is dose related but NSAIDs can cause gastrointestinal toxicity even at low doses.

Prostaglandins are important modulators of renal hemodynamics in states of reduced perfusion. Use of NSAIDs may cause a decrease in glomerular filtration rate, release of renin from the juxtaglomerular cells, increase renal vascular resistance, and redistribute intrarenal blood flow away from the papillae. This may lead to renal insufficiency with hyperkalemia and sodium and water retention.

Despite concerns about adverse reactions related to the use of NSAIDs, these drugs are effective and are the mainstay of treatment for a wide range of arthritic diseases. Acetaminophen, however, is the preferred drug for conditions where there is little inflammation and pain relief is the main objective.

Ketorolac

Ketorolac is a newer NSAID available in parenteral and oral formulations. It is soluble in water and is available as 10 mg/ml and 30 mg/ml solutions as well as 10 mg tablets. It was widely promoted for postoperative pain but reports of ketorolac-associated renal failure prompted a review of dosing regimens with a reduction in recommended doses. Patients with aspirin hypersensitivity are usually also sensitive to ketorolac, and lethal acute asthma associated with ketorolac has been reported. For these reasons, in most countries, ketorolac is not routinely used in children.

CO-ANALGESICS

There are several classes of drugs that may be used to modify or enhance the effect of simple analgesics. There is little doubt that anxiety or depression can exacerbate pain and make it difficult to treat with analgesics alone. The benzodiazepines, midazolam and diazepam, are often used in acute pain management. The tricyclic antidepressants, such as amitryptiline and doxepin, tend to be used more for chronic pain, especially neuralgias, but can be useful for short-term management of acute episodes of pain, particularly in oncology patients. Which drug is chosen depends on the individual pain experience.

Benzodiazepines

The benzodiazepines, commonly midazolam or diazepam, have several indications for use in pediatric practice as adjuncts to the simple analgesics. They provide sedation, anxiolysis, muscle relaxation and amnesia, but do not have any specific analgesic properties. They are excellent anticonvulsants. Both midazolam and diazepam are useful for premedication prior to surgery.

Midazolam is a water-soluble, short-acting benzodiazepine which has gained widespread acceptance in pediatrics. It is commonly used for its profound anxiolytic and amnesic properties and can be administered orally, intramuscularly, subcutaneously, transmucosally (rectally or intranasally), and intravenously. While it has no analgesic effects of its own, it can improve painful experiences by eliminating recall and preventing anticipation of pain.

Midazolam is a useful adjunct to both opioid and simple analgesics in the management of acute pain, such as procedural pain associated with repeated burns dressings or the regular investigations and treatment required in oncology, and for short procedures such as suturing in the emergency room (see Ch. 20) or radiological investigations. Children who are sleepy from midazolam seldom have any recall of painful procedures and are generally quiet and cooperative.

Midazolam can be titrated to effect with 0.05 mg/kg increments given intravenously. It is very potent given this way and should be administered by a medical practitioner experienced in its use. More commonly, it is given orally, 0.5 mg/kg, 30 minutes before a procedure. It may need to be mixed with a sweet drink to improve its taste. Intranasal administration of 0.2–0.3 mg/kg can be used where a more rapid onset is required or oral administration is refused. Intranasal administration causes stinging which often upsets children. Rectal midazolam, 0.75–1 mg/kg, is another alternative.

Infusions of midazolam, often combined with morphine, are commonly used for sedation in intensive care (see Ch. 19) or for reduction of distress in palliative care (see Ch. 17). Midazolam and morphine may be mixed in the same syringe. Midazolam is well tolerated subcutaneously (as is morphine).

CONCLUSION

The commonest problem with simple analgesics and sedatives is that they are underprescribed, underestimated, and not used to their potential. Careful use of these 'simple' agents will often be rewarded with good pain control with minimal complications.

4 Nitrous oxide analgesia

John Keneally

The analgesic effect of nitrous oxide was first described by Humphry Davy, in his monograph, 'Researches, chemical and physiological, chiefly concerning Nitrous Oxide', published in 1800. Davy described the pleasurable effects of inhaling the gas and suggested, 'It may probably be used with great advantage in surgical operations where no great effusion of blood takes place.' When he developed paresthesia and difficulty in concentrating, he correctly attributed these effects to the agent and they disappeared when he ceased his chronic inhalation. The intoxicating, analgesic and amnesic actions of nitrous oxide were exploited by entertainers, until Wells applied them to dentistry in 1844 and the era of surgical anesthesia truly began.

As a sole agent, nitrous oxide has been used mainly for pain relief in obstetrics, where it is self-administered via a demand valve and a close-fitting mask. Increasingly since the 1960s, a 50% mixture of nitrous oxide and oxygen (Entonox) has been utilized by ambulance services to provide analgesia to the victims of trauma and other painful conditions. Again, the gas has been self-administered via a demand valve and mask or mouthpiece, limiting its application in young children. On the other hand, constant gas flow systems, with varying nitrous oxide concentrations delivered through a nasal mask, have been widely and successfully employed by dentists in both adult and pediatric practice to produce conscious sedation and pain relief, known as relative analgesia (RA). However, the potential for nitrous oxide to provide these conditions for children during interventions such as bone marrow aspiration, lumbar punctures, venous cannulation, and wound dressings has been somewhat neglected.

ADVANTAGES OF NITROUS OXIDE

Nitrous oxide can provide both good analgesia and some sedation and amnesia, without resulting in loss of consciousness. The minimum alveolar concentration (MAC), the steady state alveolar concentration of the gas at which there is no response to surgical stimulation in 50% of subjects, is predicted to be 105% in both young children and adults.[1] Because of this relatively low potency, sudden changes in the patient's level of consciousness are unlikely when constant inspired concentrations are inhaled. Both onset and offset of action are rapid and predictable, compared with opioids, benzodiazepines and other analgesics and sedatives.

With these longer-acting agents, there is a possibility of deepening sedation once the painful stimulus is ended. In clinical use for limited periods of time, the gas has few side-effects. In healthy adults and children, cardiovascular and respiratory effects are minimal, little nausea or vomiting results, and the patient can quickly resume normal activities and feeding.

DISADVANTAGES OF NITROUS OXIDE

A number of disadvantages arise from the fact that the agent is being used to cause sedation. While, in general, the aim is to produce 'conscious sedation', there is a possibility of oversedation with consequent respiratory depression and loss of airway reflexes. During dental treatment of children, there is no suppression of laryngeal reflexes, provided the nitrous oxide concentration is adjusted to meet the individual patient's needs for analgesia.[2] However, the swallowing reflex was noted to be depressed in healthy volunteers given 50% nitrous oxide in a nonclinical situation.[3] This depression is probably no different from that caused by any other drug that results in the same degree of sedation. It is more likely to occur if the nitrous oxide is combined with other sedatives. Just as that agent has an additive effect in decreasing the MAC of other inhaled anesthetics,[1] sedatives such as opioids and benzodiazepines may markedly – and unpredictably – increase the effects of nitrous oxide. Thus, prior sedation is a relative contraindication to attempting relative analgesia unless special precautions are taken.

As nitrous oxide may increase intracranial pressure and so cause difficulty in interpreting fluctuating levels of consciousness, head injury is an absolute contraindication to the technique.

Nitrous oxide is more soluble in the blood than is nitrogen and so moves from the blood into the alveoli faster than nitrogen can be taken up in the reverse direction. If a patient is changed to breathing air immediately after prolonged nitrous oxide administration, then this difference in solubilities will mean that the concentrations of oxygen and other gases will be reduced in the alveoli. This process, 'diffusion hypoxia', can cause significant hypoxemia, and to prevent it patients must be given oxygen for several minutes. This may be difficult if Entonox has been used.

Another result of this difference in the solubilities of nitrous oxide and nitrogen is that diffusion of the former gas into air-filled spaces within the body may lead to their rapid expansion. For instance, with 75% nitrous oxide, a pneumothorax may double in size in 10 minutes. While this phenomenon is well recognized, its implications for children with asthma or other pulmonary disease often are not. In these patients, expansion of pulmonary blebs or cystic spaces may result in further derangement of lung function and, theoretically, even rupture and consequent pneumothorax. The expansion of intravascular air bubbles may be a danger in some circumstances.

The oxidization of vitamin B_{12} by nitrous oxide causes inactivation of methionine synthase and possible megaloblastic erythropoiesis. This effect is dose-related and may be worsened in patients who already have some form of bone marrow depression such as that caused by sepsis. Chronic inhalation may result in neurological effects, with subacute combined degeneration of the spinal cord – the symptoms of which Humphry Davy noticed 200 years ago. These adverse effects would not be seen in patients given nitrous oxide occasionally and for brief periods, nor have they been seen at the author's hospital, where nitrous oxide has been administered to almost all burns patients for the last 15 years. Some of these children are septic and given the gas for approximately an hour at a time, sometimes daily, for several weeks. No child has developed hematological changes attributable to this mechanism. Nonetheless, this complication is potentially serious, and regular peripheral blood studies must be conducted in such patients to detect any of its early stigmata.

The staff associated with the administration of nitrous oxide also may be at risk from prolonged exposure, unless efforts are directed at scavenging the expired gas. As well as the hematological and neurological effects, such exposure may result in a small increase in the risk of malignancy in women and may also have reproductive implications. Women dental assistants, exposed to high levels of nitrous oxide in unscavenged surgeries for more than 5 hours each week, were less than half as likely to conceive as women not exposed to the gas.[4] These occupational hazards are less likely to arise when low concentrations are used intermittently in an air-conditioned room and when active scavenging of exhaled gases is implemented.

ADMINISTRATION

Equipment

Nitrous oxide may be administered via demand units, which supply either a constant gas mixture of 50% nitrous oxide and 50% oxygen (Entonox, Fig. 4.1), or for obstetric analgesia, a nitrous oxide concentration varying from 0% to 70%. Such demand systems have the advantage that

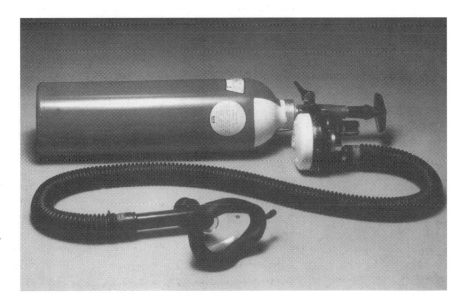

Fig. 4.1 Non-rebreathing circuit and demand valve for self-administration of Entonox (photograph reproduced with permission of Ohmeda, Australia)

they are self-administered by the patient, ensuring oversedation is almost impossible. Unfortunately, they are unsuitable for small children who may not be able to fully comprehend their use, may be unwilling to apply the mask firmly enough, or may be unable to trigger the demand valve.

Constant flow devices, such as the Quantiflex apparatus (Fig. 4.2), require the continuous presence of a qualified person, solely to administer the agent. With these machines the nitrous oxide concentration is variable to a maximum of 70%, and the gas flow ceases in the event of failure of the oxygen supply. An anesthetic machine also could be used, provided it meets standards in preventing the supply of a hypoxic gas mixture. The mask may be held by the patient or by the administrator.

Both systems require a suitable gas delivery circuit, with an exhalation valve that allows scavenging, mask or mouthpiece, and an appropriate airway filter (Fig. 4.3). Since unexpected oversedation and respiratory depression may occur, facilities and equipment for ventilation and resuscitation must be available.[5] These include:

- Staff trained in resuscitation
- A supply of oxygen and suitable devices for its administration to a spontaneously breathing patient
- A means of inflating the lungs with oxygen (e.g. pharyngeal airway, self-inflating bag)
- A trolley which can be tilted readily
- Adequate space to perform external cardiac massage
- Adequate suction and room lighting

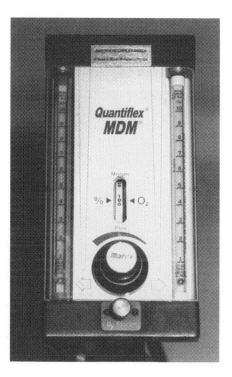

Fig. 4.2 Continuous flow, variable concentration nitrous oxide–oxygen blender (Quantiflex, Matrix Medical Inc., Orchard Park, NY, USA)

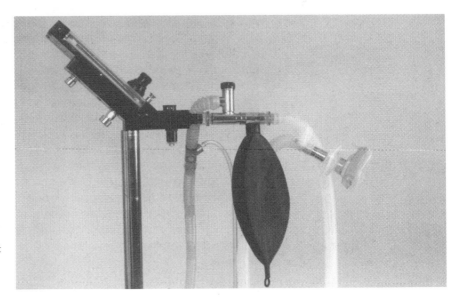

Fig. 4.3 Lightweight coaxial circuit, with airway filter, and scavenging system attached to expiratory valve (as used at the Royal Alexandra Hospital for Children, Sydney, Australia)

- Appropriate drugs for cardiopulmonary resuscitation and range of intravenous equipment
- A pulse oximeter
- Ready access to a defibrillator

Technique

Before nitrous oxide sedation or analgesia is administered, the child must be medically assessed to determine whether the technique is likely to be suitable; consent for both the procedure and the sedation must be obtained. Appropriate fasting arrangements must also be made. Those who receive any form of sedative premedication are subject to the same fasting rules as children who are to undergo general anesthesia. However, because of the low risk involved, children at the author's hospital who are to have nitrous oxide and oxygen fast for only 90 minutes.

The technique is then explained to the child in a way appropriate for his or her age. For older children using a demand system, this should include familiarization with the machine and explanation of the need to maintain a close fit with the face-mask and to take deep breaths. For either system, children should be encouraged to examine the mask and apply it to their own faces. It is important to describe the sensation of warmth in the nose and chest commonly felt as inhalation commences, and later heaviness of the limbs. It must be emphasized that the child will not be asleep and that pain will be relieved, although not necessarily abolished.

With systems that allow variable nitrous oxide concentrations, the actual administration should commence with 100% oxygen, with the mask held away from the face. This allows the patient to become accustomed to the gas flowing on to the face. The nitrous oxide concentration is then increased to about 50%. The blood and brain concentrations of the agent take 2–3 minutes to approach the inspired level and for sedation and analgesia to reach their maximum effect. No painful intervention should be allowed during that time. After this, the concentration may be altered, depending on the child's response to the stimulus. At the end of the procedure, the patient should again breathe 100% oxygen for 2–3 minutes to allow elimination of the nitrous oxide and prevent diffusion hypoxia. If any acute complications occur such as oversedation, airway obstruction, complaints of nausea, or actual vomiting, the procedure should be halted and nitrous oxide decreased or withdrawn, with extra oxygen being given until the situation is remedied.

The essential component of nitrous oxide sedation and analgesia using a continuous flow apparatus is constant and direct observation, and maintenance of verbal contact appropriate to the child's age. While a pulse oximeter should be used whenever possible (even waterproof probes are available for children having burns dressings in a bath), this monitoring is not as effective as constant, careful observation by the person administering the agent.

ADMINISTRATOR

Ideally, sedation such as that described should be given by an anesthesiologist. However, this may be impractical in a busy hospital where there is a great demand for the technique. Historically, obstetric nurses and ambulance officers have been responsible for the administration of nitrous oxide analgesia in their respective domains. This has involved self-administration by patients using demand valve systems. The administration of continuous flow, variable concentration nitrous oxide is a more vexed question, because of the greater possibility of excessive sedation. In the author's hospital, specially trained registered nurses, experienced in pediatrics and following a strict protocol developed by anesthesiologists, are allowed to carry out the majority of these procedures. Anesthesiologists are required to administer the procedure in infants less than 9 months old, those with difficult airways, patients who have been given other sedatives, or any child who is otherwise a cause for concern.

At least part of the success of this form of analgesia depends on the patience, personality and confidence of the administrator. This person must not be involved with any other part of the procedure and must have the care of the patient as his or her sole responsibility. As emphasized previously, constant careful observation of the patient and the maintenance of consciousness are paramount to the safety of the technique (Fig. 4.4).

EFFICACY

There have been a number of studies describing the use of nitrous oxide in providing analgesia and sedation for painful procedures in children. These reports describe the efficacy in a variety of situations, including minor surgical procedures and dressing changes,[6] venous cannulation,[7] and lumbar punctures and bone marrow biopsies.[8] Experience at the New

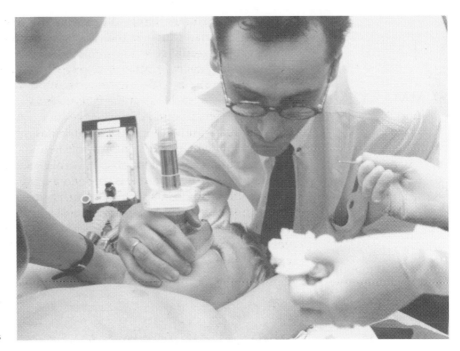

Fig. 4.4 Administration of nitrous oxide relative analgesia. The administrator's attention is focused on the patient, ensuring maintenance of consciousness

Children's Hospital, Sydney, in approximately 3000 administrations each year for such procedures, has been similarly satisfactory. The role of the technique has gradually been extended to provide sedation for investigative procedures such as nerve conduction studies, and to supplement other sedatives, for example during the more painful periods of cardiac catheterization.

Some 80% of patients experience good or excellent analgesia and about 10% some pain relief. The technique is not effective in about 10%, either because of inadequate analgesia, disorientation and dysphoria leading to lack of cooperation by the child, or (in 1–2%) nausea and vomiting. It is difficult to predict those children in whom nitrous oxide analgesia will not be successful. In some, for whom it previously has been useful, a subsequent administration may be a failure. In general, infants under 2 years old and children old enough to comprehend and cooperate are most benefited.

OTHER INHALATIONAL ANALGESIC AGENTS

Several of the volatile anesthetic agents have been used to provide sedation and analgesia. Low concentrations of trichlorethylene and methoxyflurane supplied from a drawover vaporizer have both been used for analgesia in labour. More recently, self-administered isoflurane 0.2% in nitrous oxide has been effective for obstetric pain relief.[9] Low concentrations of isoflurane used alone may be more effective in suppressing memory than MAC-equivalent concentrations of nitrous oxide, although also more potent in preventing a response to a command.[10] With reasonably rapid onset and offset of action, isoflurane thus may offer an alternative for relative analgesia, despite its irritating odour. The characteristics of sevoflurane suggest that it also may be an appropriate analgesic and sedative agent.

SUMMARY

Inhalational anesthetic agents, in particular nitrous oxide, are effective in decreasing the pain and anxiety associated with many of the painful procedures children suffer in hospital. This relative analgesia has benefits beyond opioids or other forms of sedation, and may be used to fill a gap between them and general anesthesia. The technique requires attention to detail, and must be carried out only by anesthesiologists or appropriately trained staff following a strict protocol. The establishment of a formal programme for RA allows its wide use within a hospital, with improved results and widening application as experience is gained.

REFERENCES

1. Murray D J, Mehta M P, Forbes R B, Dull D L 1990 Additive contribution of nitrous oxide to halothane MAC in infants and children. Anesthesia and Analgesia 71: 120–124
2. Roberts G J, Wignall B K 1982 Efficacy of the laryngeal reflex during oxygen–nitrous oxide sedation (Relative Analgesia). British Journal of Anaesthesia 54: 1277–1281
3. Nishino T, Takizawa K, Yokokawa N, Hiraga K 1987 Depression of the swallowing reflex during sedation and/or relative analgesia produced by inhalation of nitrous oxide in oxygen. Anesthesiology 67: 995–998
4. Rowland A S, Baird D D, Weinberg C R, Shoe D L, Shy C M, Wilcox A J 1992 Reduced fertility among women employed as dental assistants exposed to high levels of nitrous oxide. New England Journal of Medicine 327: 993–997
5. Australian and New Zealand College of Anaesthetists 1991 Policy P9. Sedation for diagnostic and minor surgical procedures. Australian and New Zealand College of Anaesthetists, Melbourne.
6. Griffin G C, Campbell V D, Jones R 1981 Nitrous oxide–oxygen sedation for minor surgery. Experience in a pediatric setting. Journal of the American Medical Association 245: 2411–2413
7. Henderson J M, Desmond G S, Komocar L J, Born G E, Stentstrom R J 1990 Administration of nitrous oxide to pediatric patients provides analgesia for venous cannulation. Anesthesiology 72: 269–271
8. Dollfus C, Annequin D, Adam M et al 1995 Nitrous oxide for providing analgesia during painful procedures required for managing pediatric malignancies. Annales de Pediatre (Paris) 42: 115–121
9. Wee MY, Hasan M A, Thomas T A 1993 Isoflurane in labour. Anaesthesia 48: 369–372
10. Dwyer R, Bennett H L, Eger E I, Heilbron D 1992 Effects of isoflurane and nitrous oxide in subanaesthetic concentrations on memory and responsiveness in volunteers. Anesthesiology 77: 888–898

5 Opioids in children

Philip Ragg

Opioids are the most frequently prescribed analgesic agents in children with severe acute pain. Advances in knowledge of the pharmacology of opioids in infants and small children and an appreciation of the need to relieve stress and pain in all children have led to the development of dosing regimens, administration techniques, and monitoring protocols that can provide children with excellent opioid analgesia safely.[1]

Historically, opioids have been underutilized in children for many reasons, often based on misconceptions and inadequate training and knowledge. It was widely believed that all children were more sensitive to opioids, that smaller infants and neonates did not feel pain, that the use of opioids for acute pain would lead to addiction, and that pain was 'character-building'. These misbeliefs implied that children had little requirement for opioids and led to a fear that they could be easily overdosed with them. Orders to administer opioids 'p.r.n.' (as required) were often interpreted to mean 'as little and as infrequently as possible'. This reluctance to administer opioids was compounded by the difficulties in assessing pain in young children and the fact that intramuscular opioids were prescribed. Children are often distressed by intramuscular injections and may deny being in pain to avoid them.[2] Finally, as infants did not remember pain and the adverse effects of pain were not appreciated, there seemed little benefit in treating pain in small children.

This chapter discusses the pharmacology of opioids, outlines how this differs between children and adults, and describes some guidelines for administration of opioids in children. Further details of monitoring and complications and their management can be found in Chapters 11 and 14.

PHARMACOLOGY OF OPIOIDS

Classification

Opioids have been classified in various ways according to their origins, structure, and actions. One classification is based on an opioid's relative efficacy (agonist, partial agonist, antagonist) at various opioid receptors. There are a number of opioid receptor subtypes including mu, delta, and kappa.[3] These receptors have multiple, often common, actions and a number of subclassifications have been described. The mu receptor is believed to have two subtypes, mu-1 and mu-2, mu-1 mediating analgesia and mu-2 respiratory depression. All clinically available opioids with action at mu receptors are nonspecific for either subtype. Mu receptors are also associated with sedation, euphoria, nausea and vomiting. Kappa receptors are associated with spinal anesthesia and sedation. Delta receptors are thought to be involved with modulation of mu receptors. Morphine, meperidine (pethidine) and fentanyl are agonists at mu receptors, buprenorphine is a partial agonist at mu receptors, and pentazocine is a partial agonist at kappa receptors. Pentazocine has a number of stimulatory actions on the central nervous system which may produce hallucinations, tachycardia, and hypertension. These effects were thought to be due to stimulation of a sigma opioid receptor. This receptor may actually be a subgroup of phencyclidine receptors rather than an opioid receptor.

Pharmacokinetics

Absorption and distribution

Lipid-soluble drugs such as fentanyl freely cross the body's membranes, which are mainly lipid, producing rapid absorption by a variety of routes and rapid distribution. After absorption into the blood stream, these drugs will quickly penetrate tissues with a rich blood supply, such as the brain. Plasma drug levels then quickly fall as lipid-soluble drugs are rapidly redistributed to large tissue depots with a poorer blood supply, such as muscle and fat. Long-term administration of these drugs will result in saturation of these tissue depots so that metabolism rather than redistribution of the drug will be required for plasma drug levels to fall. Thus, bolus doses of fentanyl for analgesia have a rapid onset and short duration of action unless the drug is given in high doses or continued for days, when its action will have a similar duration to that of morphine.

Morphine is the most hydrophilic opioid in clinical use. This results in slower passage across the body's membranes, slower uptake (if not given intravenously), and slower penetration into the brain and redistribution to other tissues. This, combined with morphine's solubility in cerebrospinal fluid (CSF), slows the onset but prolongs the duration of morphine's central nervous system effects.

Differences in lipid and water solubilities are of special importance when opioids are administered epidurally or intrathecally. Direct activation of spinal opioid receptors allows lower doses to be used, but lipid-soluble drugs will have a more rapid absorption and redistribution and therefore a relatively short duration. Morphine's solubility in CSF not only creates a depot effect producing long duration of action from small doses, but also increases the risk of profound delayed respiratory depression due to morphine migrating cephalad in the CSF. Intrathecal opioids are rarely used in children. Epidural opioids are discussed in Chapter 5.

Metabolism

Opioids (other than the short-acting agent, remifentanil) are metabolized in the liver and the water-soluble metabolites are excreted by the kidney. Morphine has an active metabolite, morphine 6-glucuronide, which has a longer duration of action than morphine but reduced potency. Glucuronidation is poorly developed in neonates but sulfation is well developed and is an alternative metabolic pathway for morphine in neonates. Meperidine is metabolized to normeperidine which may accumulate with high doses or poor renal function and cause cerebral excitatory effects including seizures.[4] Fentanyl and its analogs do not appear to have active metabolites. Morphine is the active metabolite of both diacetylmorphine (heroin) and codeine.

The bioavailability of most opioids is greatly reduced if they are administered orally. A significant proportion of the drug is metabolized by the liver, after it is absorbed from the gut, but before it reaches the systemic circulation (first-pass effect). Methadone, which has a very low plasma clearance, is an exception and has approximately 90% bioavailability by the oral route.

Pharmacodynamics

Table 5.1 lists the pharmacodynamic effects common to opioid analgesics via their action on central and peripheral opioid receptors. The spectrum of these effects will vary with different opioids, doses, and children.

Partial agonists have a lower maximum effect at the opioid receptor than full agonists. Patient variability is such that this maximum effect may be inadequate for satisfactory analgesia in some patients yet be sufficient to cause significant respiratory depression in other patients. A partial agonist acts as a partial antagonist if the child has already received a full agonist.

Although opioids have little direct effect on the heart and blood vessels, the decrease in sympathetic tone that opioids produce may cause circulatory collapse in hypovolemic patients and others dependent on high sympathetic outflow. Some opioids, such as morphine and meperidine, may cause vasodilation due to histamine release. Codeine should not be given intravenously as it may cause fatal myocardial depression by this route. Meperidine should not be used for opioid-based anesthesia for cardiac

Table 5.1 Pharmacodynamic effects of opioids

Central nervous system
    Analgesia
    Sedation
    Euphoria and dysphoria
    Nausea and vomiting
    Miosis
    Increased muscle tone (rigidity)

Respiratory
    Decreased reflex responses to hypercapnia and hypoxia
    Depression of the cough reflex
    Decreased minute ventilation (mainly by decreasing respiratory rate)

Cardiovascular
    Hypotension via depression of sympathetic tone
    Bradycardia

Gastrointestinal and urinary
    Constipation and decreased motility
    Biliary colic
    Urinary retention

Tolerance and dependence

surgery as, in the doses required, is likely to cause myocardial depression. Pentazocine may cause hypertension and tachycardia (see above).

Tolerance to opioids results in increasing dose requirements to achieve the same clinical effects. This is rare in acute pain management with opioids but may occur after several days of continuous use. High-dose intraoperative fentanyl may be associated with acute tolerance. If significant tolerance occurs the patient may become physically dependent on opioid drugs and have signs and symptoms of withdrawal if the opioids are stopped abruptly. Withdrawal may cause abdominal cramping, diarrhea, agitation, twitching, confusion and convulsions, and sympathetic activation with hypertension, tachycardia, sweating, pupillary dilatation and piloerection. Withdrawal may be managed by slowly reducing the dose, and symptom control may be aided by clonidine and central nervous system depressants. Tolerance may be managed by increasing the dose. Sensitivity to opioids has been partially restored in these patients by the use of low-dose ketamine, an N-methyl-D-aspartate (NMDA) receptor antagonist. Epidural and intrathecal opioids have also been used in oncology patients with pain in an appropriate distribution and extreme tolerance to systemic opioids.

Differences between adults and children in opioid pharmacology

The sensitivity to opioids and risk of apnea is greatest in the first 3 months of life and usually decreases to that of older children and adults by 6 months of age[5] (see also Ch. 18). Pharmacokinetic and pharmacodynamic differences in the neonate may contribute to an increased sensitivity to opioids.[5]

- Decreased liver metabolism and renal excretion and increased brain penetration may increase the risks of opioid complications such as apnea in the first weeks of life.
- Plasma protein binding of opioids is reduced in infants because of reduced binding to albumin and decreased levels of alpha-1 acid glycoprotein. This may result in more active drug being available to the tissues.

Opposing these effects is the fact that infants have a larger volume of distribution for water-soluble opioids, potentially increasing the size of required loading doses. Neonates and infants seem very susceptible to apnea due to rapid intravenous injection of morphine, most probably because their small dynamic circulation rapidly delivers a high peak blood level of morphine which penetrates the infant brain faster than the adult brain.

Infants and children in the first few years of life are less likely to vomit after opioid analgesia.

Nonpainful routes of opioid administration are preferred by children and the anticipation of an intramuscular injection may produce denial of pain.

Opioid doses in children weighing up to 50 kg should always be calculated as a dose per kilogram of body weight. Appropriately titrated adult doses can be used in larger children.

Pharmacology of specific opioid drugs

Morphine

Morphine is a mu agonist and is commonly the parenteral opioid of choice for children. It is a phenanthrene derivative with low gastric absorption and high first-pass metabolism, making its oral bioavailability less than 20%. Morphine is metabolized in the liver to the active metabolite morphine 6-glucuronide which is excreted by the kidney, and the inactive metabolite morphine 3-glucuronide which may contribute to tolerance as it is believed to have antagonist properties. Morphine causes direct histamine release which may precipitate bronchospasm, urticaria and pruritus (also believed to be centrally mediated) and vasodilatation.

The main indications for the use of morphine are analgesia and cough suppression.

Contraindications to morphine in children, as for adults, are raised intracranial pressure (unless ventilation is controlled), respiratory depression (decreased minute ventilation and/or airway obstruction), and known allergy to opioids. Relative contraindications include biliary colic, acute asthma and severe renal or hepatic dysfunction. Morphine should also be used with caution in states of hypovolemia and hypotension.

Morphine Dosage
- Bolus dose (age over 6 months)
  - 0.02–0.05 mg/kg intravenously
  - 0.5 mg/kg orally
  - 0.1–0.2 mg/kg intramuscularly every 4 hours (*Note:* intramuscular opioids are not recommended for children)
- Infusion dosage:
  - 0.01–0.04 mg/kg per hour (10–40 µg/kg per hour)

Morphine requirements may vary widely between individuals, and intravenous doses should be titrated to effect until analgesia is adequate. These dosage schedules are recommendations only, especially in the immediate postoperative period. Average morphine requirements during the first 24 hours after major surgery are 33 µg/kg per hour, with a wide standard distribution.

See Chapter 18 for a discussion of morphine administration in neonates.

Meperidine

Meperidine is a synthetic piperidine derivative and mu agonist. It has a 50% oral bioavailability. Meperidine is metabolized to normeperidine which may cause cerebral excitation, tremor, twitching, and convulsions.[4] Meperidine's pharmacodynamics are similar to morphine with a few exceptions:

- Meperidine has a shorter duration of action with single dosages (due to a greater lipid solubility).
- It gives a better treatment of shivering than other mu agonists.

The claimed decreased incidence of bronchospasm, biliary colic, and vomiting with meperidine are unproven. Both meperidine and morphine cause direct histamine release and in high doses meperidine is a cardiac depressant.

Indications and contraindications are as for morphine with the additional contraindication of concurrent or recent usage of monoamine oxidase inhibitors (MAOIs). Meperidine's interaction with MAOIs may precipitate life-threatening reactions such as hyperpyrexia, hypertension, hypotension, delirium, and seizures.

Meperidine dosage
- Bolus dose (age over 6 months)
  - 0.2–0.5 mg/kg intravenously
  - 2 mg/kg orally every 3 hours
  - 1–1.5 mg/kg intramuscularly every 3 hours (*Note:* intramuscular opioids are not recommended in children)
- Infusion dosage:
  - 0.1–0.4 mg/kg per hour (maximum 10 mg/kg in 24 hours)
  Monitor for excitatory side-effects

Codeine

Codeine is a mu opioid partial agonist. It is a phenanthrene derivative, often combined with acetaminophen (paracetamol) as an analgesic. Codeine has approximately 60% bioavailability when administered orally, with an onset time of 15–20 minutes. The clinical effects of codeine are similar to morphine but with a ceiling effect as it is a partial agonist. Codeine may cause constipation and in high doses is a cardiac depressant. Intravenous administration of codeine may cause cardiac arrest and is not recommended. Indications and contraindications for the use of codeine are as for morphine.

Codeine dosage
- Single dose – orally 0.5–1 mg/kg every 4 hours
- Intramuscular and intravenous usage are not recommended.

Fentanyl

Fentanyl is a synthetic opioid, structurally similar to meperidine, a piperidine derivative, but approximately a thousand times as potent. It is very lipid-soluble, which produces rapid onset and short duration of action unless used in high doses or for long periods (see above). Fentanyl produces minimal histamine release which improves cardiovascular stability, and is associated with a low incidence of rash and pruritus. Fentanyl inhibits central sympathetic drive so that children relying on this for cardiovascular stability may become hypotensive. Bradycardia may occur after an intravenous bolus of fentanyl. Large intravenous doses, as used in cardiac anesthesia, may produce skeletal muscle rigidity which can be controlled with nondepolarizing muscle relaxants. Unless carefully planned alternative analgesia is provided, fentanyl's short duration of action often leads to early postoperative pain

Indications and contraindications are similar to morphine. Although the risk of apnea is increased, fentanyl's short duration of action makes it useful as part of intravenous sedation techniques.

Fentanyl may be the opioid of choice in renal failure and is a useful alternative to morphine in children experiencing pruritus.

Fentanyl dosage
- Single dose – (usually intravenous) 1–2 μg/kg
- Infusion dosage – 0.5–2.0 μg/kg per hour

Alfentanil and sufentanil

Alfentanil and sufentanil are analogs of fentanyl.

Alfentanil is quite lipid-soluble and is 90% unionized at physiological pH, producing a rapid onset of action. It has a short elimination half-life and duration of action, making it ideally suited for brief painful procedures. It has a limited role in postoperative analgesia.

Sufentanil is approximately ten times as potent as fentanyl and is extremely lipid-soluble, making accumulation a problem with prolonged use. Like fentanyl it has minimal cardiovascular effect.

Neither alfentanil nor sufentanil can be recommended over fentanyl for either intravenous or epidural usage for postoperative analgesia in children.[6]

Methadone

Methadone is a synthetic diphenylheptane derivative with a long duration of action. Its action is similar to morphine. Methadone is a very effective oral opioid, having an oral bioavailability of 90%. Problems with the use of methadone include difficulties with titration of effect, and prolonged side-effects if overdosage occurs.

Dextropropoxyphene

Dextropropoxyphene is structurally related to methadone but as it is a partial agonist it has less analgesic and antitussive action. The incidence of dysphoria is higher with this agent than other opioids. It is usually administered with acetaminophen or aspirin and has a much shorter duration of action than methadone. Claims that it is less addictive have been shown to be untrue.

Indications and contraindications are as for morphine.

Dextropropoxyphene dosage
- Orally – 1–2 mg/kg every 4–6 hours.

Buprenorphine

Buprenorphine is a thebaine derivative with mixed agonist–antagonist properties. It has been shown to be effective by oral or sublingual (transmucosal) absorption. Its pharmacokinetics differ from all other opioids. It has a high affinity for opioid receptors, producing a prolonged action not clearly related to blood levels. Adverse effects may be prolonged, and naloxone may be ineffective as an antagonist of buprenorphine.

Buprenorphine dosage
- 3–5 μg/kg sublingually or by slow intravenous or intramuscular injection, every 6 hours.

Many other opioids are available but their clinical effects are similar to or have no advantage over those drugs already described. Of far greater significance in pain management in children is the route of administration.

ROUTES OF ADMINISTRATION

Opioids can be administered by a number of routes: oral, intravenous, intramuscular, subcutaneous, rectal, transdermal, transmucosal, inhalational, epidural, and intrathecal. The appropriate route will depend on patient factors (age, medical condition, past experience), surgical and medical factors (the severity of pain, type of surgery), and facilities (the location must be safe and staff and equipment suitable for the technique).

Oral, rectal and parenteral routes are the most frequently employed for acute pain management in children.

Oral opioids

The oral route of administration is very useful in children if gastric function is normal. It has the advantages that it is simple, acceptable, and risks of overdose are lower as peak blood drug levels develop more slowly.

- *Requirements*
  - the child must not be vomiting
  - the child must be able to swallow or have a nasogastric tube in situ
  - a slow onset of analgesic action should be acceptable

The oral dosage of a number of popular opioids is summarized in Table 5.2.

Table 5.2   Oral dosage of some opioid analgesics

Drug	Dose
● Codeine	0.5–1 mg/kg every 4 hours
● Morphine	0.5 mg/kg every 4 hours
● Slow-release morphine	0.2 mg/kg every 12 hours
● Oxycodone	0.2–0.3 mg/kg every 3 hours
● Buprenorphine	5 µg/kg every 6 hours
● Dextropropoxyphene	1–2 mg/kg every 4–6 hours
● Methadone	0.2 mg/kg every 12 hours
● Pentazocine	2 mg/kg every 4 hours

Rectal opioids

The rectal route of administration is potentially useful in pediatrics as it is effective if the child has gastric stasis or vomiting and it requires no special equipment. The blood supply of the rectum enables rapid absorption with higher plasma levels as first-pass metabolism may be reduced. Disadvantages of the technique are that is not accepted by some children and the drug may be expelled in feces. There is concern that neutropenic children (for example, after chemotherapy) may be at risk of sepsis secondary to bacteremia produced by placing a rectal suppository, and alternative routes should be considered.

- *Requirements*
  - no rectal or anal pathology
  - socially acceptable to family and child

Dosage regimens

- Oxycodone: 0.5 mg/kg every 8 hours
- Morphine: 0.2 mg/kg every 8–12 hours
- Codeine: 0.5–1.0 mg/kg every 6 hours

Parenteral opioids

Parenteral opioids can be administered as intermittent boluses, as continuous infusions, or as patient-controlled analgesia (see Ch. 6). As a general rule, severe pain in children is best treated with a continuous variable infusion, titrated with intravenous boluses or patient-controlled analgesia (PCA).

Intravenous opioids

The intravenous route remains the most effective and rapidly titrated method of opioid delivery. It is also the route with the greatest potential for overdosage and acute respiratory depression.[1] Children requiring continuous analgesia for moderate or severe pain are best treated with an opioid infusion or PCA. Occasionally patients may require bolus doses of opioid to cover incident pain or painful procedures such as dressing changes or removal of catheters.

Intravenous opioids should not be administered without the availability of oxygen, resuscitation equipment, and naloxone to reverse the opioid effect.

Intravenous bolus administration

The advantages of intravenous bolus administration are that it is painless and rapid in onset. The major concern with intermittent intravenous boluses is the potential for high plasma levels with subsequent respiratory depression and other complications. The potential for dosage calculation error is greater in children as opioids are given on a per kilogram basis, and dilutions, used to facilitate the administration of smaller doses, also require calculation. If an opioid infusion is in place, it can be used as the source of intravenous opioid boluses. Box 5.1 summarizes a protocol for administration of intravenous opioid boluses, including a technique for diluting the drug.

Subcutaneous opioids

The subcutaneous route is a relatively simple route of administration that can be used for intermittent boluses or continuous infusion. A cannula or butterfly needle can be placed at any convenient subcutaneous location (the clavipectoral groove is an easily accessible site). Advantages of the technique include the elimination of the need for intravenous access or repeat intramuscular injections (especially in long-term administration) and the achievement of a more constant plasma level if opioids are infused.

Disadvantages are the long onset time for boluses and long offset times if excessive effects are produced, the need for infusion equipment, and the lack of intravenous access to treat potential complications. Variability in plasma levels with changes in skin blood flow, and needle or cannula discomfort, may also be encountered. More concentrated solutions are used to minimize volumes infused. Dosage and administration are as for intramuscular opioids (see below).

Box 5.1   Protocol for intravenous opioid bolus administration

1. Before boluses are given ensure:
   a. The patient is awake and stable
   b. The intravenous line is patent
   c. The child's age and weight are known
   d. The intravenous giving set includes a burette

2. Minimum monitoring during administration should be:
   a. Pulse oximetry continuously
   b. Every 5 minutes for 20 minutes: blood pressure, heart rate, respiratory rate, and assessment of conscious state

3. The bolus dose prescription including maximum number of boluses and minimum time interval between boluses is checked. A common formula uses morphine 10 mg or meperidine 100 mg diluted to 100 ml in normal saline. The final concentration is thus 100 µg/ml morphine or 1 mg/ml meperidine. A usual bolus dose would be 0.2–0.5 ml/kg (20–50 µg/kg morphine or 200–500 µg/kg meperidine). Only the bolus dose volume should be placed in the burette.

4. The bolus dose must be administered over 5 minutes and stopped immediately if the respiratory rate or hemoglobin oxygen saturation decrease below acceptable limits.

5. After a bolus allow 5 minutes before considering another bolus.

6. If the hemoglobin oxygen saturation falls below 94% or airway obstruction or respiratory depression is suspected:
   a. Immediately stop the infusion
   b. Stimulate the patient
   c. Resuscitate as indicated including supporting ventilation
   d. Administer supplementary oxygen
   e. Consider giving naloxone (see text)

Intramuscular opioids

Advantages of the intramuscular technique include its simplicity, a slower rise in peak plasma level, and a slower onset of complications compared with intravenous administration (but more rapid than subcutaneous). Intramuscular injections are disliked by children, and some will tolerate significant pain to avoid them. Another major disadvantage is the wide intrapatient variability in analgesic effect with intramuscular opioids, which is further compounded if the pain itself is intermittent. Plasma levels will vary with conditions that alter tissue blood flow, e.g. uptake increases with anxiety and decreases with hypovolemia. Infusion catheters can be placed intramuscularly and the opioid given in the same way as a subcutaneous infusion.

Maximum recommended intramuscular or subcutaneous dosage

- Morphine: 0.2 mg/kg every 4 hours
- Meperidine: 1.5 mg/kg every 3 hours
- Buprenorphine: 5 µg/kg every 6 hours

CONTINUOUS OPIOID INFUSIONS

Compared with intermittent administration, opioid infusions produce constant plasma concentrations providing continuous analgesia. If the level of pain varies, such as incident pain, diurnal variation, or resolution of the painful condition, it is necessary to match the analgesia requirements by varying the infusion rate (up or down) or providing intermittent boluses. Alterations in infusion rate produce only slow changes in blood drug level, so boluses should be used for rapid pain control, often accompanied by an increase in infusion rate (see below).

Programmable syringe pumps or infusion devices are recommended for opioid infusions. If these devices are unavailable, it is possible to run opioid infusions using a simple bag, burette, and intravenous line system. Safety is provided by having the bag clamped off and never having more than 1 hour's dose in the burette.

Infusions can be made to varying concentrations to suit the requirements of different children, such as minimizing fluid administration after cardiac surgery. Suggested infusion protocols in either 50 ml or 500 ml dilutions are given in Appendix I. The diluent fluid is chosen to best suit the maintenance fluid requirements of the child. The total amount of intravenous fluid required per hour should be prescribed and maintenance infusions adjusted according to the opioid infusion rate. Children weighing under 10 kg will usually require more concentrated infusions than the standard 500 ml solution. Doubling the concentration (and clearly documenting this variation) or using the 50 ml dilution are satisfactory solutions. For infants less than 3 months old who are potentially more sensitive to opioids, the maximum infusion rate prescribed should be half to three-quarters of the usual maximum (20–30 µg/kg per hour for morphine) and the initial infusion rate not more than half the usual maximum (20 µg/kg per hour for morphine). Opioid infusions in neonates are discussed in Chapter 18. These patients require close observation, including pulse oximetry (see also Ch. 11).

Breakthrough pain or inadequate analgesia

Problems of inadequate analgesic are also discussed in Chapter 14.

If a child on an opioid infusion requires increased analgesia, this can be done by administering a bolus of opioid (usually the same dose given in 1 hour at the previous infusion rate) and turning up the infusion rate. For example, a patient on 20 µg/kg per hour opioid infusion of morphine experiencing continuous pain should be given a single bolus of 20 µg/kg (i.e. the previous hourly infusion rate) and the infusion rate should be increased to 30 µg/kg per hour. If the infusion rate alone is increased without a bolus dose being given, it will be some hours before the plasma level will rise and the child may unnecessarily remain in discomfort for this period. If multiple boluses are required and the maximum infusion rate is being used, occasionally children will require higher infusion rates. Monitoring should be increased if this occurs. In older children, PCA may provide better analgesia.

For children receiving opioid infusions it is important that the nursing staff are sufficiently trained so that a prescription of morphine of up to 40 µg/kg per hour, with boluses of 20 µg/kg per hour with a minimum of 10 minutes between boluses, can produce 'nurse-controlled analgesia' of similar quality and safety to PCA.

Complications

A more detailed discussion of the management of complications of opioids can be found in Chapter 14 but some problems particularly related to infusions are discussed here. Good management of complications such as nausea and vomiting may allow adequate analgesic dosage to be tolerated.

Overdosage may occur due to dose calculation error, failure to match decreasing analgesia requirements with decreasing infusion rates, the slow rise in blood drug concentrations that occurs over several hours after an increase in infusion rate, or a change in pharmacokinetics such as occurs when a child becomes hypovolemic. Close supervision and monitoring (see Ch. 11) of children receiving opioid infusions are important, as appropriate doses for analgesia in an awake child may produce apnea when the child is asleep.

If multiple intravenous infusions are connected to a single intravenous cannula, care must be taken to avoid problems with opioid passing backwards into another infusion system and then being flushed into the patient. A one-way valve in the other line can prevent this problem. The opioid infusion should be attached close to the patient to prevent flushing of large amounts of opioid if the other infusion has intermittent flow.

Care must be taken to decrease opioid infusions as the patient's requirements decrease. Alternative analgesia, usually oral, should be continued or introduced to minimize opioid requirements. Opioid analgesia may assist mobilization, but if continued longer than necessary can delay mobilization. After major abdominal surgery, younger children usually require opioid infusions for 1–2 days rather than the 2–3 days often required by older children.

NEW ROUTES OF ADMINISTRATION

Newer routes of opioid administration, such as transdermal patches with slow release of lipid-soluble opioid such as fentanyl, transmucosal 'lollipops' for analgesia or premedication such as oral transmucosal fentanyl citrate (OTFC), and intranasal sprays, are currently being evaluated.[7]

The transdermal route has variable absorption, a long onset time (12–18 hours) and a slow fall in plasma concentration on removal.[7] This makes its usefulness better suited to longer-term analgesia such as cancer pain. The incidence of side-effects such as nausea, vomiting, and respiratory depression are similar to parenteral routes, and plasma levels are more variable and often low.[8] Analgesia provided by these routes often requires supplementation.

NALOXONE

Naloxone is a pure opioid antagonist at mu, delta, and kappa receptors. It is nonselective and will antagonize all the effects of opioid receptor stimulation including analgesia, respiratory depression, and sedation.[9] This may cause withdrawal in patients receiving long-term opioid therapy. Complications of naloxone include acute pain (due to antagonism of analgesia) tachycardia, hypertension, tachypnea, arrhythmias, cardiac failure, and pulmonary edema. Careful titration of naloxone can avoid most of the complications due to the stimulation resulting from reversal of analgesia, but pulmonary edema may be an idiosyncratic complication, not related to dose or stimulation.

Naloxone is rapidly eliminated and has a shorter duration of action than most opioid analgesics. If a patient is successfully treated with naloxone, monitoring should continue to ensure that the adverse opioid effects do not reappear with the rapid decline in naloxone blood levels. If repeated doses are required, a naloxone infusion may be safer than intermittent boluses. Less easily titrated but potentially useful for a longer duration of action is the use of intramuscular naloxone.

It is important to note that a patient found to be apneic needs immediate restoration of respiration. If stimulation does not produce an immediate response, artificial ventilation should be commenced, the pulse checked, and basic resuscitation instituted. These activities should take priority over administering naloxone (see below).

Naloxone dosage

Give 2–10 μg/kg intravenously as a bolus and repeat, doubling the dose until clinically effective up to 100 μg/kg, then repeat as required. If repeated doses are required, an infusion may be commenced at 1 μg/kg per hour and titrated to effect.

If intravenous access is not available naloxone may be administered intramuscularly, subcutaneously, or via the intraosseous route. The intramuscular and subcutaneous doses are 5–10 μg/kg. Both these routes have slower onset (subcutaneous is the slower) than the intravenous route, and a longer duration of action. The intraosseous dose is the same as the intravenous dose.

MANAGEMENT OF RESPIRATORY DEPRESSION

Mild respiratory depression

Mild respiratory depression is defined as a moderate decrease in the respiratory rate, with the hemoglobin oxygen saturation decreased but greater than 90%.

- *Management:*
  – consider decreasing or ceasing opioid if associated with marked sedation
  – administer oxygen
  – stimulate the patient
  – continuously monitor pulse oximetry, heart rate, and respiratory rate

Severe respiratory depression

Severe respiratory depression is defined as apnea, HbO_2 saturation less than 90%, or a significant decrease in respiratory rate *or* heart rate.

- *Management:*
  – support airway, breathing and circulation (ABC) as required
  – stop opioid administration

- administer oxygen
- give naloxone 2 µg/kg up to 100 µg/kg intravenously, titrated by doubling the dosage as required
- summon the resuscitation team
- continuously monitor pulse oximetry, heart rate, respiratory rate, and blood pressure

CONCLUSION

Opioids are effective analgesics which can be administered to children of all ages. Careful titration of dose to the child's needs, close monitoring (Ch. 11), adequately trained staff, and prompt management of complications (Ch. 14) are required for safety and to maximize the efficacy of these drugs. For other opioid-related techniques see Chapters 6 and 7.

Note: Sample opioid prescription forms may be found in Appendix I. These were designed for use in the Royal Children's Hospital, Melbourne, Australia. These forms take into account the training, accreditation, and resuscitation facilities at that hospital and are likely to need modification for use in other institutions.

REFERENCES :

1. Lloyd-Thomas AR 1990 Pain management in paediatric patients. British Journal of Anaesthesia 64:85–104
2. Mather M, Mackie J 1983 The incidence of postoperative pain in children. Pain 15:271–282
3. Shipton E 1993 Primary analgesics. In: Shipton E (ed.) Pain acute and chronic. Witwatersrand University Press, Johannesburg, ch 2 pp. 29–47
4. Armstrong P, Bersten A 1986 Normeperidine toxicity. Anaesthesia and Analgesia 65: 536–538
5. Brown TCK, Fisk GC 1992 Paediatric anaesthetic pharmacology. In: Brown TCK, Fisk GC (eds) Anesthesia for children, 2nd edn. Blackwell Scientific, ch 2, pp. 25–52
6. Chrubasik J, Wust H, Schulte-Monting J, Thon K, Zindler M 1988 Relative analgesic potency of epidural fentanyl, alfentanyl and morphine in treatment of post operative pain. Anaesthesiology 68:929–933
7. Gaukroger P 1993 Novel techniques of analgesic delivery. In: Schecter N, Berde C, Yaster M (eds) Pain in infants, children and adolescents. Williams & Wilkins; Baltimore, pp. 195–200
8. Mather L 1991 Novel methods of analgesic drug delivery. In: Bond M, Charlton J, Woolf C (eds) Proceedings of the VIth World Congress on Pain. Elsevier, Amsterdam, Ch 18, pp. 159–173
9. Yaster M, Deshpande J 1988 Management of paediatric pain with opioid analgesics. Journal of Pediatrics; 113:421–429

6

Patient-controlled analgesia

Phil Gaukroger

INTRODUCTION

Patient-controlled analgesia (PCA) is widely used for the management of many forms of acute pain in both adults and children. The pharmacological and psychological advantages of allowing patients to control their own pain relief have been well demonstrated.

The term PCA usually refers to the intravenous administration of small bolus doses of an opioid on demand to treat acute pain. The patient has a hand-operated device which, when activated, triggers the machine to deliver a bolus into the patient's intravenous line provided that a set period of time (lockout interval) has elapsed since the previous dose. The lockout interval allows the previous dose to take effect before another dose can be delivered, and prevents potential overdose.

THE BENEFITS OF PCA

The advantages of PCA include a high degree of patient satisfaction owing to the psychological benefits of 'control'. The technique allows for wide variability in individual opioid requirements, avoids delays in analgesic administration, reduces nursing staff workload and, when properly prescribed and supervised, provides the greatest degree of safety of any method of systemic opioid delivery.

The use of PCA in pediatric care reduces the need for negotiation between the child and the staff and prevents the possibility of conflict if further analgesia is not forthcoming. Older children may be able to titrate a balance between analgesia and side-effects such as sedation, nausea and vomiting, and pruritus. Most patients do not attempt to achieve total analgesia but are willing to tolerate some pain with the knowledge that it will not become overwhelming and that they can quickly control it. Adolescents appreciate the benefits of 'control' more than younger children.

PATIENT SELECTION

Patient-controlled analgesia is suitable for all types of acute pain in children old enough to manage the technique. It is most commonly used for postoperative pain following major general, thoracic, or orthopedic surgery. Children with burns, cancer, and other types of longstanding acute pain can also benefit from PCA.

Initial fears regarding the ability of children to responsibly control their own opioid therapy have been unfounded. The technique can be used by any child who is able to understand the concept of PCA and who is able to work the apparatus.[1,2] Most children 7 years and older will use PCA well. Children 4–6 years old may be better managed with conventional opioid infusions or other nurse-administered techniques, but some can use PCA effectively if adequately instructed preoperatively and encouraged postoperatively.

What should children be told about pain and PCA? It is important to ensure that the child's expectations are realistic. Children benefit from honest explanation of how much pain they are likely to experience postoperatively so that they can prepare themselves for the postoperative course. They need explanation of how the PCA machine works and how the lockout interval works, and they need to know that pain is not eliminated but rather brought down to a manageable level. Suitable, honest explanation is one of the most important factors in reducing anxiety and is often ignored in children.

DRUG PRESCRIPTION IN PCA

Morphine is a suitable drug and is most commonly chosen for PCA in children, although a wide range of agents can be used. In general, mu agonists are used for PCA. Partial agonists are not as suitable, having a lower maximum analgesic effect. Many centers restrict the use of meperidine (pethidine) for PCA because the high doses that may be administered have occasionally produced normeperidine toxicity even in patients without renal impairment. Some devices can be programmed to limit the maximum dose delivered, in which case a maximum of 10 mg/kg per 24 hours is usually prescribed for meperidine. If higher doses are required an alternative opioid, usually morphine, can be used. Fentanyl is also a useful alternative and is less likely to produce pruritus.

Doses for pediatric PCA are prescribed according to the child's weight. Most pediatric hospitals find it convenient to vary the amount of opioid added to the syringe (according to weight) and keep the volume of doses constant, rather than reduce the volume of the bolus dose. This becomes important for safety reasons as the bolus dose volume in most PCA systems should be at least 0.5 ml. Most pediatric anesthesiologists calculate opioid doses in μg/kg and should know how many μg/kg of opioid are in each milliliter of their institution's standard PCA dilution. Arithmetically simple dilutions are easily understood and increase safety. For example, as commonly used for morphine, 0.5 mg/kg in 50 ml equals 10 μg/kg per ml, or 1.0 mg/kg in 50 ml equals 20 μg/kg per ml.

Commonly used PCA settings for morphine in children are as follows:

- Bolus dose 15–20 μg/kg
- Lockout interval 5 minutes
- Background infusion (when used) : 5–15 μg/kg per hour.

Most PCA equipment requires the doses to be prescribed in micrograms or milligrams. To simplify prescription and minimize calculation and preparation errors, it may be helpful to draw up a prescription chart for the different opioids that are used. A standard dose per kilogram of opioid (e.g. 1.0 mg/kg morphine, 10 mg/kg meperidine or 20 μg/kg fentanyl) is put in 50 ml, the concentration produced is calculated (required for setting the PCA device) and a standard volume bolus (usually 1 ml for the concentrations just mentioned) and background (0.5–1.5 ml/h) if required, is prescribed. Some centers further simplify the calculations by having standard prescriptions for patients within 5 kg weight ranges as illustrated by Tables 6.1, 6.2 and 6.3 for morphine, fentanyl, and meperidine, resectively.

Table 6.1 Morphine PCA prescribing chart

Weight of child (kg)	Syringe order (mg/50 ml)	Bolus dose (mg)	Lockout interval (min)	Concentration (mg/ml)	Background infusion (mg/h)
50	50	1.0	5	1.0	0.5
45–49	45	0.9	5	0.9	0.45
40–44	40	0.8	5	0.8	0.4
35–39	35	0.7	5	0.7	0.35
30–34	30	0.6	5	0.6	0.3
25–29	25	0.5	5	0.5	0.25
20–24	20	0.4	5	0.4	0.2
15–19	15	0.3	5	0.3	0.15

Table 6.2 Fentanyl PCA prescribing chart

Weight of child (kg)	Syringe order (μg/50 ml)	Bolus dose (μg)	Lockout interval (min)	Concentration (μg/ml)	Background infusion (μg/h)
50	1000	20	5	20	10
45–49	900	18	5	18	9
40–44	800	16	5	16	8
35–39	700	14	5	14	7
30–34	600	12	5	12	6
25–29	500	10	5	10	5
20–24	400	8	5	8	4
15–19	300	6	5	6	3

Table 6.3 Meperidine PCA prescribing chart. Meperidine administration should be restricted to 10 mg/kg per 24 hours to prevent normeperidine toxicity.

Weight of child (kg)	Syringe order (mg/50 ml)	Bolus dose (mg)	Lockout interval (min)	Concentration (mg/ml)	Background infusion (mg/h)
50	500	10	5	10	5
45–49	450	9	5	9	4.5
40–44	400	8	5	8	4
35–39	350	7	5	7	3.5
30–34	300	6	5	6	3
25–29	250	5	5	5	2.5
20–24	200	4	5	4	2
15–19	150	3	5	3	1.5

The PCA settings may need to be modified for children who have developed tolerance to opioids, such as some oncology patients. Bolus size may need to be increased and background infusions may reduce demands and prevent withdrawal symptoms.

Background infusions are usually omitted in adult practice. Their use in pediatric practice remains controversial. Possible benefits of adding a background opioid infusion to PCA in children include better pain control, especially in the prevention of episodes of sleep disturbance and awakening in severe pain. Possible disadvantages of adding a background infusion to PCA in children are that opioid consumption and side-effects such as nausea and vomiting are greater, that safety is compromised (opioid delivery continues despite sedation or respiratory depression), and that pain relief is often no better.

Background infusion doses are also controversial. Some centers routinely use low-dose (morphine 5 µg/kg per hour) background infusions, reserving higher doses (morphine 15 µg/kg per hour) for opioid-tolerant patients. Other centers will have wider indications for the higher doses, particularly when severe pain will occur, such as in the first days after major spinal, thoracic, or abdominal surgery. Indications for background infusions include:

- Major surgery (first 1–2 days)
- Burns
- Oncology
- Other opioid-dependent patients
- Younger children

When a background infusion is used for major surgery or in other children whose opioid requirements are decreasing, it is appropriate to reduce or omit the infusion after 24–48 hours. If excessive side-effects are experienced, the initial management should be to remove the background infusion.

RECOVERY ROOM AND WARD MANAGEMENT

In children undergoing surgery, an adequate loading dose of morphine (usually 0.2 mg/kg) is best given intraoperatively so that the child arrives in the recovery room in a comfortable state and severe pain is avoided. If short-acting drugs such as fentanyl are used for intraoperative analgesia, more severe pain may be experienced in recovery as the duration of action of fentanyl is very short in children. Pain in the recovery room should be prevented rather than treated and the most suitable way is to adequately load the patient intraoperatively with the opioid that will be used postoperatively. Clinically, it seems to be more difficult to control pain once the patient is awake than if adequate analgesia is given intraoperatively.

Children receiving PCA should usually have hourly nursing observations. Observations consist of pulse rate, respiratory rate, volume delivered, and simple assessments of pain, sedation, and nausea and vomiting, using verbal rating scales. Pulse oximetry should be used continuously in high-risk patients and available for spot checks if there is suspicion of respiratory problems in other patients (see below and Ch. 11).

Supervision of children using PCA can be undertaken by either the ward staff looking after the patient or shared with an acute pain management service. The prescribing and programming of PCA must be undertaken by staff experienced in the area, usually anesthetic personnel. Other physicians, such as the clinician in charge of the patient's main surgical or medical condition, should be suitably trained before attempting to prescribe PCA. A team approach is required, with the anesthesiologist or pain management team assisting rather than competing with the other physicians in the management of the patient.

PARENTS AND PCA

The role of parents during PCA in children should be considered. Parents can be helpful in providing encouragement and support to children in the postoperative period. They need to be told that for reasons of safety their child must be the only person to use the PCA button.

Parents can reinforce the concept of PCA with the child before surgery and help to consolidate the information already provided to the child about PCA. They are often at the child's bedside during the postoperative phase and can, if required, assist by reminding the child to press the button if a painful incident is forthcoming or if the child appears to be in significant pain.

COMPLICATIONS

Up to one-third of children will experience opioid-related side-effects while on PCA (see also Ch. 14). Persistent nausea or vomiting can be managed with intravenous metoclopramide or ondansetron in addition to reassessing the child's pain and PCA settings. Consideration should be given to reducing opioid requirements by adding acetaminophen (paracetamol) or a NSAID. For children in whom vomiting is a greater problem than pain it is desirable to omit the background infusion and allow them to balance their nausea and pain. Occasionally, changing to a different opioid is effective.

Sedation – either excessive or too little – appears to be a minor problem with PCA. Urinary retention is no more common than with intramuscular opioids. Pruritus can occur in up to 20% of children on intravenous morphine and is troublesome in about 5%. Changing to fentanyl PCA is usually effective, and is a simpler option than administering antihistamines or small doses of naloxone.

Respiratory depression due to opioid PCA is potentially the most dangerous side-effect but rarely has serious consequences. The reliance on patient activation and small boluses makes severe respiratory depression unlikely. The safety of PCA in children has been well supported by the very few cases of respiratory depression that have occurred despite widespread use of pediatric PCA. Approximately 1% of pediatric patients using PCA (most often adolescents) have respiratory rates of less than 10 breaths per minute. This is usually managed by stopping the PCA for a period and administering oxygen if associated with hemoglobin desaturation. Some of these children may have had drug interactions with sedating antihistamine or antiemetic drugs. Naloxone is rarely required as respiratory depression is usually mild.

Safety with PCA is ensured by having only the child activate a bolus. Even if errors occur in the setting of bolus dose size or concentration, a wide range of doses will be tolerated by the child who can compensate by changing the frequency of demands for a bolus. Properly prescribed PCA is one of the safest methods of administering opioid analgesia in children.

Oxygenation

Research in the adult population has found a high incidence of desaturation episodes during the postoperative period in patients receiving opioids. One study of 75 children using PCA demonstrated 84% of SpO_2 readings were in the range 95–100% only 1% of SpO_2 recordings were less than 90%, and none was associated with slow respiratory rate or sedation.[3] Another study of 19 children showed no significant change in oxygen saturation before and after surgery, and postoperative oximetry in a further 50 children requiring systemic opioids or epidural analgesia demonstrated a mean saturation of 97.8% ($\pm$ 1.9% SD).[4] These data suggest that, in contrast to adults, most children do not have multiple episodes of significant oxygen desaturation in the postoperative period. Clinically, this implies that there is no need for the routine administration of oxygen to children postoperatively.

Pulse oximetry should be available for spot checks in wards where children have undergone major surgery. Continuous pulse oximetry is usually reserved for children who have undergone surgery that is expected to impair respiratory function, or who have significant preoperative cardiorespiratory impairment (see Ch. 11).

ALTERNATIVE ROUTES OF ADMINISTRATION

The subcutaneous route may be used for PCA in patients requiring longer-term opioid analgesia who do not have intravenous access and who find the oral route of drug administration ineffective or intolerable. Compared with intravenous administration, the speed of onset and offset is slower. Itching and redness at the site of insertion and pain during the administration of subcutaneous PCA doses may bother some children. The bolus dose should be increased to at least 50 µg/kg and the lockout interval increased to 20 minutes because it takes longer to reach peak blood levels and effects. Children suitable for subcutaneous PCA are often tolerant of opioids, so drug consumption may be high. To reduce the volume of the bolus dose, the concentration of opioid should be increased so that the amount received per hour is unlikely to exceed 0.5 ml. Apparatus suitable for administering small volumes must be used. Morphine and hydromorphone are the most suitable drugs for subcutaneous use because they are less likely to be irritant than meperidine, and because they are available in more concentrated forms.

Epidural PCA has been described in both adults and children. While most of these small studies have reported favorably on the technique, considerable work is awaited in this area. Appropriate bolus dose settings, lockout intervals, and background infusion rates have not yet been determined. Many investigators are unsure whether pain relief from epidural PCA opioids is any better than from intravenous administration.

SPECIAL APPLICATIONS

The technique of PCA is particularly useful for children who experience recurrent or long-term pain such as those with burns,[5] cancer, or requiring palliative care. These children are very appreciative of the 'control' which is afforded to them by PCA. These applications are discussed in Chapters 16 and 17.

EQUIPMENT

The majority of PCA machines are designed for bedside use and have battery back-up which allows them to be used during transportation. Recently, a number of PCA devices for ambulatory patients have become available. These devices are compact, portable, and usually battery-powered.

The ability to program smaller bolus doses is necessary with children and when using potent drugs such as fentanyl. Weights of children able to use PCA vary from 15 kg upwards, and the smaller patients will require bolus doses of as little as 0.25 mg of morphine.

Hand-control design has received little attention in relation to children using PCA, although small children have successfully used a wide variety of hand controls. A pneumatically operated button (Graseby, Watford, UK) may have advantages for children unable to use their hands (such as those with burns or those born without upper limbs), in that the device can be easily modified to allow foot operation. Pneumatic buttons can also be exposed to water in the bath or a bed without suffering damage.

The ability to program a background infusion is an advantage for children but is not available on all machines. Devices should be tamper-proof to prevent use by siblings and other children in the ward, and to prevent the stealing of drugs from the machine.

Attention must be paid to the safety of the intravenous delivery system for PCA, especially if the intravenous line used for PCA is shared with other infusions. Many centers use infusion pumps and syringe drivers for all intravenous fluid delivery in children. These devices prevent backflow and will sound an alarm if obstructed. If a gravity-driven infusion shares the line with a PCA infusion, there is a risk that obstruction distal to the junction of the infusions can result in the PCA delivering opioid backwards into the other line. If the obstruction is then cleared, the opioid collected in the other line may be delivered as a dangerous bolus. Placing a one-way valve in the gravity-fed line before it is joined by the PCA line should prevent this complication. The PCA line should join the other line close to the intravenous catheter to minimize the dead space to be filled and the volume that might be flushed if flow in the other line is intermittent. A separate intravenous cannula used solely for PCA will prevent these problems, but may not be practical in some children.

CONCLUSION

Patient-controlled analgesia is a suitable method for providing pain relief to the majority of school-aged children experiencing both short-term and longer-term acute pain. Putting patients in control of their own pain relief clearly distinguishes this method from other methods of opioid administration, and accounts for the high degree of satisfaction experienced by both patients and parents. The technique also offers benefits in terms of staff time and safety which are not possible with other methods of intravenous analgesia. It is now an accepted technique for the control of acute pain in school-aged children and its use in pediatric institutions is widespread and increasing.

Note: A sample prescription form and a protocol for the use of PCA may be found in Appendix II. These were designed for use in the Royal Children's Hospital, Melbourne, Australia. These forms take into account the training, accreditation and resuscitation facilities at the hospital and are likely to need modification for use in other institutions.

REFERENCES

1. Gaukroger PB, Tomkins DP, Van der Walt JH 1989 Patient-controlled analgesia in children. Anesthesia and Intensive Care 17:264–268.
2. Gaukroger PB 1993 Patient-controlled analgesia in children. In: Schechter N, Berde CB, Yaster M (eds) Pain management in children and adolescents. Williams and Wilkins, Baltimore, pp. 203–211.
3. Morton NS 1993 Development of a monitoring protocol for safe use of opioids in children. Pediatric Anaesthesia 3:179–184.
4. Tyler DC, Woodham M, Stocks J et al. 1995 Oxygen saturation in children in the postoperative period. Anesthesia and Analgesia 80:14–19.
5. Gaukroger PB, Chapman MJ, Davey RB. Pain control in pediatric burns – the use of patient-controlled analgesia (PCA). Burns 17:396–399.

7

Epidural analgesia in children

Philip Ragg

INTRODUCTION

Epidural analgesia has become a well-established method of pain relief in neonates, infants, and children, for a number of reasons. Equipment specifically designed for pediatric epidural blockade has been developed. The understanding of the physiology and pharmacology of epidural analgesia in children has improved. The quality of analgesia attainable with epidural techniques has encouraged hospital staff and helped fulfill the increasing expectations of patients and their families for good pain relief. The advent of acute pain management services has provided the support required for epidural analgesia to become a routine technique in many centers.

Analgesia following major surgery of the trunk or lower limbs is the most common indication for epidural catheterization. It is usually performed after induction of general anesthesia. Several advantages of epidural anesthesia and analgesia have been proposed. Intraoperative epidural anesthesia may decrease the amount of general anesthetic and opioid drugs required, enabling early extubation, awakening, feeding, and (in neonates) bonding. Operating conditions may be improved by the contracted bowel and decreased blood loss[1] associated with epidural blockade. Analgesia may be better than with other techniques. Epidural infusions may be continued for some days, usually until analgesia can be managed with simple oral agents.[2] Outcome may be improved with lower morbidity rates, especially respiratory complications.[3]

This chapter covers lumbar and thoracic epidural analgesia in children, but not caudal epidural blockade (see Ch. 8) or intrathecal analgesia.

ANATOMY AND PHYSIOLOGY

Younger children have body proportions differing from those of adults, having a relatively greater body surface area, shorter limbs, and a larger head.[4] Ligaments are thinner and bones softer, which may make landmarks for epidural injection more difficult to identify.[5] The depth of these landmarks varies with age and size (see below). The anatomy of the midline and paramedian approaches to the epidural space are shown in Figure 7.1 (see below for a description of the method of insertion). Pharmacological differences influence selection of drug dose and concentration. Local anesthetic

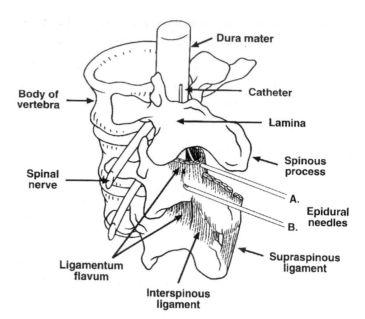

Fig. 7.1 The anatomy of the midline (A.)and paramedian (B.) approaches to the epidural space. See text for further details

agents have greater volumes of distribution in children, which will decrease the blood levels associated with initial doses. Neonates have decreased clearance of local anesthetic drugs compared with older children, limiting the infusion rates that they will tolerate. Protein binding of local anesthetic drugs is lower in the first year of life (lower levels of alpha-1 acid glycoprotein and albumin), increasing the proportion of free drug in plasma. Myelination is incomplete in infants[4] and the nodes of Ranvier are closer together, potentially making these nerves more susceptible to local anesthetic blockade. The sympathetic nervous system is not mature at birth and side-effects due to sympathetic blockade such as hypotension are uncommon in children less than 8 years old.[6]

The level of the dural sac and spinal cord change during infancy. In the full-term neonate, the dural sac extends to the third or fourth sacral segment (S3–4) and the spinal cord to the fourth lumbar vertebra (L4). At 6 months of age the dural sac is at S2 and the spinal cord at L2–3. By 1 year, the dural sac and cord are at adult levels, S1 and L1 respectively.[4] Surface anatomy landmarks are also different in neonates and infants. The intercristal line (joining the iliac crests) crosses the midline at L5–S1 in neonates, at L5 in children and at the L4–5 interspace in adults. The scapula tip is usually at T7 as in adults.[4] The epidural space in infants contains nerve roots, fat, lymphatics, and blood vessels as in adults, but the structures are loose, enabling catheters to traverse the space more readily.[7]

The approximate depth of the epidural space in infants (less than 10 kg) and children can be estimated from their body weight (*Wt*) in kilograms, using the following formula for the average distance (*d*) in millimeters from skin to ligamentum flavum.

- Infant: $d = 1.5 \times Wt$
- Child: $d = Wt$

For example, the average depth of the ligamentum flavum of an 8 kg infant can be calculated as follows:

$$d = 1.5 \times 8 = 12 \text{ mm}$$

These formulae are a guide only, and insertion techniques should allow for a more superficial epidural space in some children.

PREPARATION FOR EPIDURAL BLOCKADE IN CHILDREN

For the safe performance of any central neural blockade technique in children, careful preparation and selection of the patient and equipment and appropriately trained staff are required.

Location

Epidural insertion is usually performed under general anesthesia in children and must therefore be performed in an appropriate location. All equipment required for monitoring, maintenance, and recovery must be available and suitable for the age of patient. Resuscitation drugs and equipment necessary for the management of epidural complications and side-effects must be immediately available.

Assistance

As patient monitoring cannot be maintained alone during insertion of an epidural, a trained assistant must be present and attending the patient at all times.

Intravenous access

Intravenous access must always be established prior to epidural insertion. Reliable access must be maintained until cessation of the epidural blockade. Fluids for resuscitation must be available.

Equipment

Equipment for the performance of an epidural blockade must be prepared with a sterile technique. Materials needed are listed in Box 7.1. A sterile epidural kit will usually contain the components listed in Box 7.2.

Box 7.1 Equipment for epidural insertion

Sterile gloves
Sterile drapes and swabs
Antiseptic solution
Tray or table
Needles and syringes (single use only)
Tapes and dressings
Local anesthetic solution
Epidural kit (see Box 7.2)

Choice of needle

Needles used for epidural analgesia in children include 19 gauge, 18 gauge, and 16 gauge diameters. Although controversy exists as to the relative merits of these narrower needles in smaller children, it is likely that

---

Box 7.2   Epidural kit

Needle (Tuohy or curved bevel)
Catheter
Filter
Loss of resistance syringe
Connector

---

the smaller the diameter the less trauma is done to ligaments and, should dural tap occur, the smaller the leak of cerebrospinal fluid (CSF).

Epidural needles for children should have an inner stylet (to prevent coring of tissue), a rounded, short, directional bevel (as in a Tuohy needle), a single end hole, and gradations on the side (0.5 or 1 cm) commencing at the tip.

As a general guide to size for age or weight, 19 gauge needles are suitable for children up to 20 kg (age approximately 5 years) and 18 gauge needles are used for children 20 kg and upwards (5 years to teenage). Although 19 gauge needles may be suitable for older children, their use is limited by their short length (5 cm) and the inability of some pumps to deliver clinically required flow rates through the small (23 G) high-resistance catheter used with this needle.

Epidural catheters

Epidural catheters should be the largest appropriate for the needle used (Table 7.1) and should meet as many of the criteria for an ideal epidural catheter (Box 7.3) as possible.

Table 7.1   Epidural needle and catheter gauge

Needle gauge	Catheter gauge
20	24
19	23
18	20

Box 7.3   Properties of an ideal epidural catheter for children

Clearly marked with cm lines
Firm but not so stiff as to cause trauma
Tensile strength (enabling safe removal)
Made of inert material (no tissue reaction)
Kink resistant
Smooth, round, atraumatic tip
Radiopaque

Catheters of 23 G and 24 G have a single end hole as it is technically difficult to produce them of such fine gauge with side holes and guarantee integrity. The higher incidence of occlusion compared with larger catheters probably relates to kinking of the finer catheter, rather than the absence of side holes. Smaller catheters sometimes have a stylet for stiffness to facilitate threading. Markings should be in centimetres, with a double mark at 10 cm and a triple mark at 15 cm, as on larger catheters. Earlier pediatric catheters had a double line at 5 cm, creating confusion.

Filters and connectors   Low dead space, lightweight connectors and filters are preferable in children. Most bacterial filters in common pediatric usage have a 0.2 μm pore diameter.

Indications

Epidural analgesia for children is suitable for most painful procedures or trauma involving the trunk, thorax, abdomen, pelvis or lower limbs, i.e. any major procedure involving dermatomes T5 to S5. Specific examples include thoracic, abdominal (fundoplication, operations for Hirschsprung disease), genitourinary (reimplantation of ureters, pyeloplasty, hypospadias repair), and orthopedic (lower limb and pelvic) surgery. Epidural analgesia may be indicated for prevention of specific complications of surgery, such as bladder spasm after urological procedures, skeletal muscle spasm after surgery in children with cerebral palsy, and incident pain with coughing after thoracotomy. Microvascular free flaps may have enhanced graft blood flow with epidural induced sympathetic blockade.[3] Epidural analgesia may also be indicated in children sensitive to the side-effects of opioids, for example those with limited respiratory reserve, and in children undergoing surgery where control of pain with opioids may be difficult.

The surgical indications for epidural analgesia at the Royal Children's Hospital in Melbourne over a 4-year period are summarized in Figure 7.2. The age distribution of epidural usage for this period is shown in Figure 7.3.

Contraindications

Contraindications to epidural analgesia are listed in Box 7.4. Some of the contraindications to epidural usage in children are relative and a decision should be made as to the risks versus the benefits of the technique for an individual patient. Epidural analgesia may still be appropriate in the presence of a relative contraindication (e.g. bacteremia) if there are strong contraindications to alternative analgesia, or strong indications for epidural analgesia.

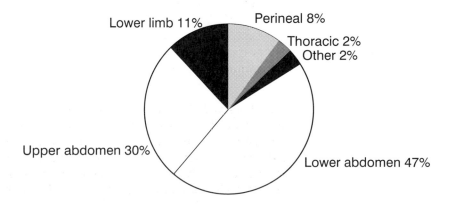

Fig. 7.2 The frequency of various surgical indications for epidural analgesia in children at the Royal Children's Hospital, Victoria, Australia

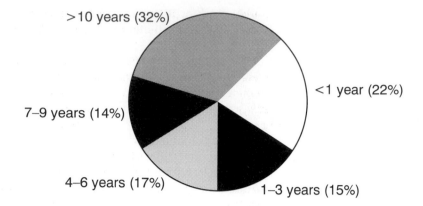

>10 years (32%)

<1 year (22%)

7–9 years (14%)

4–6 years (17%)

1–3 years (15%)

Fig. 7.3 Age distribution of children having epidural analgesia at the Royal Children's Hospital, Victoria, Australia

TECHNIQUE OF INSERTION

General principles

Appropriate preparation (see above) before an epidural catheter is inserted in any child includes obtaining informed consent and intravenous access, and checking the equipment. The practitioner performing the epidural blockade should be suitably trained or supervised. Children are usually anesthetized prior to its insertion. The catheter is usually inserted with the child placed in the lateral position, and surface landmarks (see above) should be identified. The tip of the epidural catheter should ideally be located in the middle of the dermatomal spread required.

Insertion of needle and catheter

The back is prepared with bactericidal solution, using gloves and an aseptic technique, and drapes are placed to create a sterile field. Precautions that should be taken with epidural needles in children include supporting the needle at all times, estimating the distance expected to the epidural space prior to insertion (remembering that bone and ligaments are soft and can easily be penetrated), ensuring the stylet is at the end of the needle, never forcing a needle, never withdrawing catheters through needles, and disposing of needles carefully.

With the desired level of insertion chosen, either a midline or paramedian technique (see Fig. 7.1) is commonly performed to identify the epidural space.

Box 7.4   Contraindications to epidural analgesia

Absolute

    Coagulopathy
    Inadequate facilities or staffing
    Lack of consent
    Raised intracranial pressure
    Infection over the site of insertion

Relative

    Bacteremia
    Cardiovascular impairment
    Progressive neurological deficit

The midline approach involves identifying the interspinous space and slowly advancing the Tuohy needle in the midline. During this maneuvre it is helpful for the assistant to put counterpressure on the abdomen so that the child does not move away from the operator. Little resistance should be encountered until the ligamentum flavum is entered. At all times attention must be given to the distance and direction the needle has travelled. A 'loss of resistance' syringe should be connected when either the ligamentum flavum is encountered or the estimated distance to the ligament has been reached. To connect the syringe, remove the stylet and continue to support the needle with one hand, as the needle may easily fall out of the ligament. Slowly advance the needle and syringe, using gentle, continuous pressure on the plunger; a distinct decrease in resistance should be felt when the epidural space is entered (compared with complete loss of resistance in the adult). Immediately immobilize the needle and support it as the syringe is disconnected. Care must be taken to inject only a small volume of air or saline. The 'hanging drop' or balloon techniques for identifying the epidural space are more difficult in children as the tissues are softer. Aspirate and observe for dural tap or intravascular insertion. The catheter should now be advanced, making note of the distance of the needle tip to the epidural space. Catheters are usually advanced 2–5 cm into the epidural space. Secure the catheter as described below. Before any injection of local anesthetic solution, an aspiration test should be performed to ensure no blood or cerebrospinal fluid enters the catheter.

The paramedian technique[8] involves advancing the epidural needle just lateral to the spinous process at the desired level. With the thumb on the appropriate spinous process the needle is advanced perpendicular to the back at 90 degrees to the skin, parallel to the midline, beside the spinous process. The needle may be 'walked' down the lateral side of the spinous process to the lamina, or aimed directly at the lamina. When the lamina is located, the needle is walked cephalad off the bone into the ligamentum flavum. The technique is otherwise the same as the midline approach. Supporters of this approach claim the use of the bony landmarks allows more certainty in locating the depth of the ligamentum flavum.

Loss of resistance

Loss of resistance syringes for identifying the epidural space may be used, containing either gas (usually air, but carbon dioxide is recommended by some to decrease the consequences of gas embolism) or liquid (usually saline). There is a difference in the 'feel' of the loss of resistance with gas or liquid and most anesthesiologists will have a preference for the feel of one or other method. The incidence of air embolism is decreased with saline[9] but the diagnosis of dural tap is more obvious with air. 'Missed segments' of nerve block and neurological damage have been ascribed to air injection in the epidural space. Whichever method is used, a minimum amount of the content of the loss of resistance syringe should be injected when the loss of resistance is felt.

The level at which the epidural catheter is inserted is dependent on the anesthesiologist's experience and preference. While it is agreed that the tip of the catheter should finish at the middle dermatome of the region to be blocked, controversy exists as to the relative merits of threading catheters from the caudal canal or inserting them directly into the thoracic or lumbar space. The caudal route is accepted in many centers for use in infants weighing less than 10 kg.[10] An end-hole needle, rather than a Tuohy needle, may increase the success rate of threading catheters from the caudal canal to the lumbar or thoracic epidural space.

While the field is sterile, the catheter connector junction should be checked to ensure that it is firm yet allows injection. Disconnection or occlusion at this junction are common problems if this is not checked at this stage. Needles and sharps should be appropriately disposed of before ungloving.

Fixation of the catheter

Children are often very active, especially when comfortable, so securing the catheter well at the time of insertion is important. A clear occlusive dressing reinforced with tape around the edges ensures that the entry site through the skin is visible and local reactions can be diagnosed. Flexible nonocclusive dressings (e.g. Hypafix) are also well tolerated by children. A loop of catheter under these dressings gives a margin for catheter movement on the skin without dislodging it from the epidural space. Taping the catheter all the way up the back (without tension on the tape and with the back flexed, to prevent the catheter migrating out later), then bringing it over the patient's shoulder and taping the padded bacterial filter and connector to the chest, is often convenient, comfortable, and secure.

CHOICE OF LOCAL ANESTHETIC SOLUTIONS

Single shot or intraoperative local anesthesia

Considerations in choosing the type of local anesthetic solution used intraoperatively include speed of onset, duration of action, dose, and concentration.

Onset and duration of action

Agents such as lidocaine (lignocaine) or prilocaine, with a rapid onset of action, are useful for emergency surgery or acute orthopedic trauma. Longer-acting agents such as bupivacaine and ropivacaine provide better postoperative analgesia after a single dose.

Dermatomal spread

There is considerable patient variation, but the following formula can be used as a guide to the volume of local anesthetic solution required:

Volume in ml of local anesthetic solution per dermatome blocked = (age in years)/10

The actual dose of local anesthetic agent in mg/kg should be calculated from the volume and concentration used to ensure that it is within the maximum recommended dose. To minimize the volume of local anesthetic solution required, the catheter should be placed with the tip at the dermatome in the centre of the area producing the pain stimulus.

Concentration of local anesthetic drug

More concentrated solutions usually produce greater muscle relaxation. For bupivacaine, 0.125% usually produces little motor block, 0.25% often produces motor block, while 0.5% will usually produce marked motor block. Equivalent concentrations of lidocaine are 0.5%, 1% and 2% respectively. Bupivacaine 0.25% is usually used intraoperatively and 0.125% for postoperative epidural infusions.

Epinephrine

The addition of epinephrine (adrenaline) 1 in 200 000 (5 µg/ml) may increase the duration of action of epidural bupivacaine, especially in younger children.[11] This is believed to be due to local vasoconstriction and decreased vascular uptake of the agent. Epinephrine addition may also be useful for the detection of intravascular injection if a test dose is given while monitoring the heart rate. This is less reliable in the anaesthetized child.

Continuous infusions of local anesthetic solution

Similar considerations as for single shot techniques apply to continuous infusions, but the duration of action is less critical as a constant supply of local anesthetic drug is available. However, the development of tachyphylaxis is a major disadvantage of lidocaine, so most centers use bupivacaine. Often motor blockade is not desirable postoperatively, so more dilute concentrations of local anesthetic agent will produce analgesia (sensory blockade) without decreased mobility. Hypotension secondary to sympathetic blockade is uncommon in younger children.[2]

A recommended commencement regimen for epidural infusions in children is 0.2 ml/kg per hour of 0.125% bupivacaine (range 0.1–0.3 ml/kg per hour). Suggested maximum doses of bupivacaine are outlined in Table 7.2. The 'initial bolus' to establish the block will usually be given in the operating room, often in increments, and rarely will require more than 2 mg/kg. The top-up bolus doses are suggested for inadequate block when less than the maximum infusion rate is being used. Bupivacaine 0.125% is frequently used, but a 0.25% solution may be used if a more profound block in similar dermatomes is required (see also 'Management of inadequate epidural blockade' below).

The long half life of bupivacaine in neonates and younger infants means that plasma levels produced by an epidural infusion may still be rising on the second postoperative day. To minimize the risk of local anesthetic toxicity,[12–14] infusions are usually discontinued earlier in these smaller patients. Fortunately, the duration for which epidural analgesia is required is generally shorter in younger children. Consideration should be given to cessation of the infusion at 24 hours for infants less than 6 months old, at 36 hours for children aged 6–24 months, and at 48 hours for

Table 7.2 Recommended maximum epidural bupivacaine dosages. These recommendations refer to patients who will have continuation of epidural blockade via a catheter. Bolus injection should be avoided in patients receiving the maximum infusion rate

	Age <6 months	Age > 6 months
Initial bolus (mg/kg)	2	2.5
'Top-up' bolus (mg/kg)	0.25	0.4
Infusion (mg/kg per hour)	0.25	0.4

children aged 2–10 years, and it is uncommon for any postoperative epidural analgesia to be required beyond 72 hours. Usually, when the epidural infusion is stopped, the catheter is not removed until it is clear that simple oral analgesia will provide good pain control.

Other possible reasons to terminate an epidural infusion in children include signs of infection (local or systemic), failure of analgesia, suspected intravascular or subarachnoid migration of the catheter, significant leakage around the catheter insertion site, or contamination of the catheter by accidental disconnection or dislodgement. (See Ch. 11 for further discussion and protocols for monitoring and safe management of epidural infusions in children.)

ADMINISTRATION AND PREPARATION OF EPIDURAL INFUSIONS

Any epidural delivery system must be closed to prevent contamination and accidental administration of drugs not intended for the epidural space. An accurate means of delivering a set volume or infusion rate is required, e.g. a syringe pump. An example of such a system is shown in Figure 7.4.

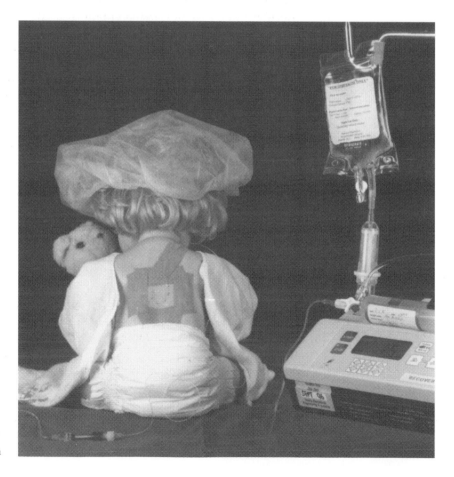

Fig. 7.4   The epidural system

Epidural solutions must be clearly marked and catheters clearly labeled, and all care taken to avoid accidental injection or addition of substances not intended for the epidural space. Suggested strategies include not having injection ports in the epidural delivery system or covering them with tape. Training of staff is most important as a preventive measure in this area. Ideally, epidural solutions containing several drugs (e.g. opioid and local anesthetic) should be standardized and supplied sterile by the hospital pharmacy using either commercial or in-house preparations. Anesthesiologists must use meticulous sterile techniques if making up these solutions themselves.

Epidural opioids

Epidural opioids are often added to local anesthetic regimens to improve the quality of analgesia.[15] They do not cause sympathetic or motor blockade.

The choice of epidural opioids includes hydrophilic and hydrophobic agents. Hydrophilic drugs such as morphine have a long duration of action due to slow CSF elimination. Morphine may have an action at sites distant from the local epidural site due to cephalad spread. Lipophilic opioids such as fentanyl and meperidine (pethidine) have a more rapid onset of action, shorter duration, and an action closer to their site of administration.[8] A suggested delivery regimen is to add fentanyl 2 μg/ml to bupivacaine 0.125%. The recommended range of infusion rates of 0.1–0.3 ml/kg per hour would deliver 0.2–0.6 μg/kg per hour of fentanyl.

The potential complications of epidural opioids in children are summarized below. Early respiratory depression is more common with lipid-soluble opioids such as fentanyl. This respiratory depression is due to rapid systemic absorption and is usually mild, as the dose used epidurally is low. Delayed respiratory depression is probably due to slow rostral migration of opioid in the CSF.[16] This may produce sudden apnea without a prodrome of worsening respiratory depression. This is more likely with the more hydrophilic morphine. Pruritus is also more common with epidural morphine than with fentanyl.[3] Both pruritus and respiratory depression may be treated with naloxone 5–10 μg/kg intravenously; however, opioid analgesia may also be reversed by naloxone.

MANAGEMENT OF INADEQUATE EPIDURAL ANALGESIA

A careful history and thorough examination of the child should be performed when inadequate analgesia is reported. This should include determining the onset, character, and consequences of the pain, and assessing the child's vital signs and state of hydration. Pain after surgery may be a sign of a new medical or surgical problem and consultation with medical colleagues may be indicated. An assessment (see below) must be made to ascertain whether modification of the epidural block is likely to provide analgesia. If this seems likely, the steps outlined below should be followed. See Chapter 14 for further general discussion of the management of inadequate analgesia.

Assessment of epidural blockade

Satisfactory adjustment of an inadequate epidural block is more likely if there is a history of good analgesia in the early postoperative period than if the block has never been satisfactory. The trend of pain scores should be noted. An attempt should be made to define the extent of sensory blockade. This may be extremely difficult in young or developmentally delayed children. Cold or light touch can be used to map the dermatomal spread of the block. Unilateral blockade or blockade that is above or below the painful site may be demonstrated. The efficacy of analgesia can also be checked by assessing the ability of the child to breathe deeply, change position, or cough.

Management of inadequate epidural blockade

Check the delivery system

Drug: Is the right drug being delivered, at the correct concentration, volume and rate?

Catheter: Check that the catheter is not disconnected, kinked, leaking excessively, intravascular, subdural, or out of the epidural space.

Modify the block

1. For unilateral or too high a block, withdrawing the catheter (if sufficient catheter is in the epidural space) may improve the block.
2. Lie the patient in an appropriate position to allow gravity to assist reestablishment of the blockade.
3. Give a bolus of epidural solution to reestablish a block that is unilateral, too high, or too low. Bolus doses are usually reserved for patients on less than the maximum infusion rate. Doses are as in Table 7.2. Inadequate dermatomal spread can be treated by giving a bolus of 0.125% bupivacaine and increasing the infusion rate. A block of the correct dermatomes but inadequate potency can be treated with a 0.25% bupivacaine bolus. This may be accompanied by increasing the concentration of the infusion while maintaining the rate, provided the dose is within the recommended maximum. Appropriate observations should be commenced after any bolus or increase in rate (see Ch. 11).
4. Consider changing the epidural solution. Options include adding an opioid, increasing the concentration of local anesthetic, increasing the volume or rate of infusion, removing epidural opioids, and adding another systemic analgesic .
5. If the epidural continues to be unsuccessful, order an alternative analgesic or reinsert the catheter. The latter is rarely done as most children would require either sedation or general anesthesia for insertion of another epidural catheter, and alternative analgesia is usually acceptable.

If the pain appears unrelated to the surgical wound (e.g. shoulder tip pain or headache after pelvic surgery), consideration should be given to adding another analgesic such as acetaminophen (paracetamol) or a nonsteroidal antiinflammatory drug. An intravenous opioid infusion could be used if there is no opioid in the epidural infusion. The use of systemic opioids with epidural opioids is contraindicated because of the significant risk of respiratory depression. There is controversy about when it is safe to commence systemic opioids once epidural opioids have been stopped. If fentanyl has been infused epidurally in the doses described above (0.2–0.6 μg/kg per hour) and the patient has inadequate analgesia, the practice at the Royal Children's Hospital, Melbourne, is to stop the epidural fentanyl and commence intravenous morphine as required. If the patient had received epidural morphine (which is not usually given via an epidural catheter) prolonged intensive monitoring would be essential if an intravenous opioid was required. The combination of intravenous opioid and epidural local anesthetic drugs may not only produce satisfactory analgesia but may also provide a degree of sedation and anxiolysis that will smooth the general management of the child. Suitably trained nursing staff can titrate the opioid infusion as required (see Ch. 5).

COMPLICATIONS OF EPIDURAL ANALGESIA IN CHILDREN

The complications of epidural analgesia in children can be divided into three groups:

1. Technique problems (Table 7.3)
2. Drug-related problems (Table 7.4)
3. Catheter problems (Table 7.5)

A number of these complications are discussed in more detail in Chapter 14.

Table 7.3 Epidural analgesic in children: problems of technique

Problems	Comments	Treatment
● Headache	May be due to dural tap (incidence 1–2%) Uncommon in children < 8 years old	1. Analgesia 2. Bed rest 3. Fluids 4. Epidural blood patch if prolonged, typical postural headache
● Backache	At insertion site Usually transient	Simple analgesics and reassurance
● Sympathetic blockade	May cause hypotension (usually in children older than 8 years)	1. Posture (lie flat) 2. Intravenous fluids (10 ml/kg) 3. Vasoconstrictors
● High blockade	1. Respiratory distress (intercostal block) 2. Bradycardia (high thoracic block) 3. Unconsciousness (total spinal block)	1. Resuscitation 2. Cease epidural infusion 3. ? Recommence at lower dose if epidural position confirmed
● Nerve damage	Very rare May present weakness or numbness Usually transient	1. Investigation 2. Neurology referral 3. Review
● Bleeding or infection	Very rare Presents with back pain, fever, sensory or motor deficit. *Note:* 'At risk' patients (eg. abnormal coagulation, immunosuppression)	1. Urgent investigation 2. Neurology referral

Table 7.4   Epidural analgesia in children: drug-related problems

Problems	Comments	Treatment
Local anesthetic drugs		

● Intravascular injection	May be minimized by:
	    aspiration test
	    test dose
	    safe dosing levels
		1. Stop the infusion
		2. Remove the catheter
		3. Resuscitate as necessary

● Overdose	Signs of local anesthetic toxicity may be present	Resuscitation and management of cardiac, neurological and respiratory side-effects
● Allergy	Extremely rare Signs of anaphylaxis or allergic reaction may be present	Resuscitation, intravenous fluids, adrenaline, antihistamines and steroids
Opioids		
● Respiratory depression	Early or delayed.	1. Oxygen/Resuscitation 2. Naloxone 3. See protocol in Ch. 5
● Nausea and vomiting	More common with morphine than fentanyl	1. Antiemetics 2. Consider cessation of opioid
● Pruritus	More common with morphine than fentanyl	1. Anti-histamines 2. Topical calamine and cooling techniques 3. Intravenous naloxone
● Urinary retention		1. Conservative methods (see Ch. 14) 2. Urinary catheter
● Reactivation of herpes simplex	Rare in children	

Table 7.5   Epidural analgesia in children: catheter-related problems

Problems	Comments	Treatment

● Leakage	Incidence approximately 6%
	Less likely with:
	    subcutaneous tunneling of the catheter
	    paramedian technique.
		1. Gauze pad and pressure dressing
		2. Topical solutions (e.g. compound benzoin tincture) at the skin insertion site to cause contraction of the skin around the catheter

● Occlusion or kinking	Approximately 11% of catheters occlude or kink	1. Check the catheter and the system 2. Overcome with bolus 3. Change the infusion rate
● Dislodgement	About 5% of catheters disconnect Prevent with meticulous connection and dressing at time of insertion	Check connections regularly Remove catheter if disconnection occurs

CONCLUSION

Epidural analgesia is a specialized technique and, as for all pain management methods, the potential benefits must be weighed against the risks. It can provide excellent, safe analgesia for children of all ages when performed and supervised by adequately trained staff.

Note: A sample prescription form and a protocol for epidural analgesia may be found in Appendix III. These were designed for use in the Royal Children's Hospital, Melbourne, Australia. These forms take into account the training, accreditation, and resuscitation facilities at that hospital and are likely to need modification for use in other institutions.

REFERENCES

1. Johansson K, Ahn H, Lindhagen J 1988 Effect of epidural anesthesia on intestinal blood flow. British Journal of Surgery 75:73–76
2. Dalens B, Tanguy A, Haberer J 1986 Lumbar epidural anesthesia for operative and postoperative pain relief in infants and young children. Anesthesia and Analgesia 65:1069–1073
3. Liu S, Carpenter R, Neal J 1995 Epidural anesthesia and analgesia. Anesthesiology; 82:1474–1506
4. Brown TCK, Fisk GC 1992 Anesthesia for children, 2nd edn. Blackwell Scientific, London
5. Saint-Maurice C, Schulte-Steinberg O 1990 Regional anesthesia in children. Mediglobe, Fribourg, pp. 18–20
6. Murat I, Delleur M, Esteve C, Egu J, Raynaud P, Saint-Maurice C 1987 Continuous extradural anesthesia in children. British Journal of Anesthesia 69:1441–1450
7. Ecoffey C, Dubousset A, Samii K 1986 Lumbar and thoracic epidural anesthesia for urologic and upper abdominal surgery in infants and children. Anesthesiology 65:87–90
8. Cousins M, Bridenbaugh P 1988 Neural blockade, 2nd edn. JP Lippincott, Philadelphia
9. Sethna N, Berde C 1993 Venous air embolism during identification of the epidural space in children (editorial) Anesthesia and Analgesia 76:925–927
10. Bosenberg A, Bland B, Schulte-Steinberg O, Downing J 1988 Thoracic epidural anesthesia via the caudal route in infants. Anesthesiology 69:265–269
11. Warner M, Kunkel S, Offord K, Atchison S, Dawson B 1987 The effect of age, epinephrine, and operative site on the duration of caudal analgesia in pediatric patients. Anesthesia and Analgesia 66:995–998
12. Luz G, Innerhofer P, Bachmann B, Frischhut B, Menardi G, Benzer A 1996 Bupivacaine plasma concentration during continuous epidural analgesia in infants and children. Anesthesia and Analgesia 82:231–234
13. Larsson B, Olsson G, Lonnquist P 1994 Plasma concentrations of bupivacaine in young infants after continuous epidural infusion. Pediatric Anesthesia 4:159–162
14. Berde C, 1992 Convulsions associated with pediatric regional anesthesia. Anesthesia and Analgesia 75:164–166
15. Wilson P, Lloyd Thomas A 1993 An audit of extradural infusion analgesia in children using bupivacaine and diamorphine. Anesthesia 48:718–723
16. Lloyd-Thomas AR 1990 Pain management in pediatric patients. British Journal of Anesthesia 64:85–104

8 Caudal epidural analgesia

Ian McKenzie

INTRODUCTION

Caudal epidural injections of local anesthetic solution produce analgesia that may be useful for procedures up to the umbilicus. The height of the block will depend on the volume injected, while the degree of sensory and motor block depends on the concentration used. The dose of local anesthetic drug must be carefully calculated to ensure that the dose per kilogram is within safe limits for that patient. More peripheral nerve blockade may be an alternative to caudal injection. Some centers use infusions of local anesthetic solution via caudal epidural catheters to prolong postoperative analgesia.

The caudal route has been used to place catheters with their tip at lumbar or thoracic levels.[1] The effect of local anesthetic drugs injected at these sites is described in Chapter 7. There is controversy over both the reliability of catheter placement (especially in older children) and the risk of infection if the catheter is left for postoperative pain control. Various spinally active analgesics, such as opioids and clonidine, can be administered by the caudal route, but they have their own complications and their clinical place is evolving.

ANATOMY

The distal end of the spinal canal is the sacrococcygeal membrane (Fig. 8.1). The sacral portion of the canal has sacral bodies anteriorly, and sacral

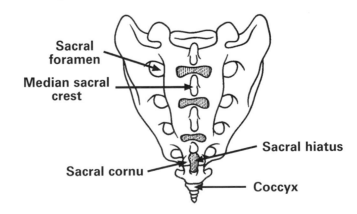

Fig. 8.1 Posterior view of the sacrum. The sacrococcygeal membrane covers the sacral hiatus. The degree of posterior bony fusion varies between patients and with development

spines (median crest) and lamina posteriorly. The sacrococcygeal membrane forms the posterior wall of the caudal end of the spinal canal, lying distal to, and sometimes continuing cranially between, the sacral cornua. Just deep to this membrane lies the epidural space. This is the site of caudal epidural injections. It is located by palpating the sacral cornua. In the adult, this is often deep in the natal cleft. In neonates and infants the pelvis and buttocks are relatively smaller, and the sacral hiatus is usually well above the natal cleft. The site of the sacral hiatus usually forms the apex of an equilateral triangle with its base the line joining the 'dimples of Venus', indentations of the skin over the sacroiliac joints, just medial to the posterior superior iliac spines (Fig. 8.2). The use of these landmarks to locate the cornua will overcome the common error of those more familiar with the adult anatomy who tend to look too low for the sacral hiatus in infants. If coccygeal structures are mistaken for sacrum, the needle may be passed between coccygeal segments into the pelvis. Perforation of the rectum has occurred.

Ossification of the sacrum continues throughout childhood. The success rate of caudal injections (though still high) is lower in children over 8 years old.[2] The relative softness of the sacrum in young children increases the chance of penetrating the anterior wall of the sacral canal, potentially leading to the equivalent of intravascular injection into the bone marrow. Incomplete sacral ossification allows a 'transsacral' interspinous approach,[3] analogous to interspinous epidural injections as used in the lumbar region, to be used as an alternative route to the caudal canal in children.

In older children, the dural sac usually ends at the level of the body of the first sacral segment. In neonates, the dural sac usually ends at the third sacral segment. Sacral anatomy varies between patients, so that if a low dural sac is combined with a high sacrococcygeal membrane (in some variants of spina bifida the posterior sacrum may not fuse), dural puncture is more likely. Alternatively, fusion of the posterior sacrum may be nearly complete, almost obliterating the sacral hiatus.

The sacral portion of the spinal canal has a substantial epidural venous plexus. Careful avoidance of intravenous injection (see below) is of prime importance for safe caudal anesthesia.

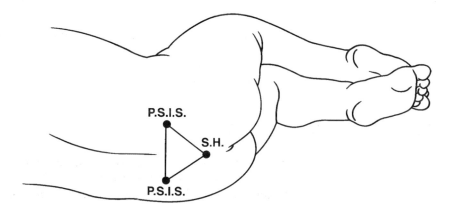

Fig. 8.2 Child positioned for caudal blockade by a right-handed anesthesiologist. Surface landmarks of sacral hiatus are highlighted. PSIS, posterior superior iliac spine; SH, sacral hiatus

TECHNIQUE

Caudal injections in children are usually given with the patient in the lateral position after induction of general anesthesia. The anesthesiologist must be satisfied that the patient's airway is being safely maintained and that suitable monitoring is in place while the block is performed. The usual contraindications for regional block apply (see Ch. 7), such as local infection or coagulopathy. Sterile technique must be used. If there is fecal soiling, the region should be thoroughly washed prior to the application of antiseptic solution. Right-handed anesthesiologists generally prefer the patient positioned left side down, allowing the right hand to advance the needle while the left thumb defines the apex of the sacrococcygeal membrane, without crossing hands.

Except where there is marked failure of fusion of the posterior sacrum, the sacrococcygeal membrane should be punctured at its apex (cranial end). The membrane is thickest at this point, giving a more obvious 'pop' or loss of resistance when punctured. As the anteroposterior depth of the canal decreases distally, apical puncture makes it easier to place the whole tip of the needle in the canal without encountering the anterior wall. The needle should be advanced gently to increase appreciation of penetration of the sacrococcygeal membrane and minimize the risk of penetration of the anterior wall of the sacral canal. The needle is commonly advanced at an angle of about 60 degrees and should be stopped as soon as the canal is entered. The practice of then decreasing the angle and advancing the needle up the canal increases the risk of vascular or dural penetration. The anteroposterior dimension of the sacral canal is small in neonates and infants. Placement of the needle tip within the shallow sacral canal of these young patients may be easier if the skin is penetrated caudal to the sacral hiatus and the needle advanced at an angle of 45 degrees or less.

In infants and neonates a small (e.g. 24 gauge) intravenous cannula may be used for caudal injections. After penetration of the sacrococcygeal membrane the stylet is partially withdrawn and the cannula slid up the sacral canal. The method described above where the needle is inserted distally and advanced almost parallel with the sacral canal decreases the risk of the catheter kinking. This technique enables placement of the solution, careful testing that the injection is extravascular (see below), and minimal trauma, with confidence that small movements of the catheter tip are less likely to enter vessels or damage tissue than needle tip movements.

Correct placement of a needle for caudal epidural injection is associated with minimal resistance to injection, no sign of subcutaneous swelling on injection, and no evidence of blood or cerebrospinal fluid on aspiration or disconnection of the syringe.

DRUGS, DOSAGE AND INDICATIONS

Bupivacaine is the drug most commonly used. Its slow onset is a minor disadvantage as caudal anesthesia in children is mostly combined with general anesthesia, although some anesthesiologists use a mixture with lidocaine (lignocaine) to speed onset. The long duration of action of bupivacaine is a major advantage when prolonged postoperative pain relief is required. This may be prolonged by the use of epidural infusions via catheters in appropriate cases.

With sufficient volume of local anesthetic solution, caudal analgesia can be used in procedures up to the umbilicus. It is especially suitable for perineal and penile procedures. Inguinal and umbilical surgery are also suited to local field blocks and local infiltration which will avoid some of the complications specific to caudal analgesia. The reliability, ease of performance, remoteness from the surgical site, and preoperative timing of caudal anesthesia can make it preferable to these alternatives. In neonates and infants having inguinal surgery, the landmarks for ilioinguinal blockade may be difficult to feel, making caudal anesthesia more attractive.

Selection of an appropriate volume and concentration of local anesthetic solution for pediatric caudal analgesia has been a source of some confusion. Some anesthesiologists use 1 ml/kg of 0.25% bupivacaine as a universal caudal dosage. This is simple, but will often result in significant leg weakness which may delay discharge in older patients. A dose of 2.5 mg/kg is conservative compared with the 3 mg/kg maximum commonly quoted in pediatrics, but still above the 2 mg/kg maximum recommended by the product information in many countries. Higher doses of bupivacaine (with epinephrine (adrenaline)) have been used uneventfully in children,[4-6] but 3 mg/kg is normally the maximum clinical dose. Many formulae for calculation of pediatric caudal doses have been suggested.[7,8] Each patient's requirements should be considered individually. An appropriate volume of local anesthetic solution for the desired height of the block and concentration for the required density of blockade should be selected according to the guidelines below. Before injection, the dose per kilogram should be calculated to ensure that it is safe.

A dose of 1 ml/kg of caudal local anesthetic solution will usually block up to the lower to middle thoracic level, 0.5 ml/kg to the midlumbar level, and 0.2 ml/kg the sacral segments (saddle block). Bupivacaine 0.25% produces surgical anesthesia and moderate motor block. If residual motor block is a contraindication to discharge from day surgery (which is not the case in all centers), a weaker solution can be used for day patients. Bupivacaine 0.125% has been recommended[9] but deeper general anesthesia is often required owing to its weaker intraoperative effects, and a few patients will have inadequate analgesia postoperatively. These factors may delay discharge, which is earliest when 0.175% bupivacaine is used.[10] An alternative approach to obtain good intraoperative conditions yet avoid leg weakness, for outpatient penile procedures in children old enough to walk, is to use 0.15–0.2 ml/kg of 0.5% bupivacaine. For inpatient hypospadias procedures 0.5 ml/kg of 0.5% bupivacaine will give a dense block of long duration, the motor block being a potential advantage in the early postoperative phase.

For major hypospadias repairs, pelvic surgery such as low anastomosis for Hirschsprung disease and orthopedic procedures on the lower limbs where there will be a need for prolonged postoperative analgesia, a caudal catheter may be used. Standard pediatric epidural kits and infusion regimens may be used (see Ch. 7). The dressing must be waterproof to avoid fecal soiling, and the catheter exit from the dressing should be well away from the anus. Alternatively, transsacral or low lumbar epidural catheters can be used. These move the insertion site further from the anus but increase the chance of dural puncture. Most infusions can be stopped by 48 hours, and should rarely continue beyond 72 hours postoperatively.

A published dose regimen of caudal bupivacaine as an alternative to spinal or general anesthesia for 'high-risk, ex-premature' infants having inguinal hernia surgery under local anesthesia alone is 3.25 mg/kg of bupivacaine 0.2% with epinephrine 5 μg/ml.[4,11] Good general management of the patient is vital to the success of the technique. Secure intravenous access, monitoring of oximetry, electrocardiography, noninvasive blood pressure and temperature, firm wrapping of the upper trunk and arms, leg restraints, availability of a pacifier ('dummy') that may be coated with 50% dextrose solution, and waiting at least 10 minutes after the block before surgery starts are all important.

ADDITIVES AND OTHER DRUGS

The use of epinephrine with bupivacaine in children is controversial. The usual concentration used is 5 μg/ml (1 in 200 000). Peak local anesthetic blood levels after single injection caudal blockade are approximately halved by the addition of epinephrine.[5,12] This improves the safety margin, but recommended doses of bupivacaine without epinephrine already have an excellent safety record. Epinephrine may assist in the detection of intravascular injection but is not completely reliable (see below), and may increase the risk of life-threatening ventricular arrhythmias if a major intravenous injection of local anesthetic drug occurs. The theoretical risk of ventricular arrhythmias due to the interaction of halothane, hypercarbia (from spontaneous ventilation anesthesia) and epinephrine (added to the caudal local anesthetic solution) has not been a significant clinical problem in children.

There is conflicting evidence about whether children have a substantially longer duration of analgesia if epinephrine is added to bupivacaine.[13,14] Epinephrine may prolong bupivacaine caudal analgesia more in younger children.[13] Confusion has also arisen from the fact that the prepackaged 'with epinephrine' solutions are of lower pH (about 5) than solutions that have epinephrine added by the operator (pH about 6.5). The lower pH may adversely affect onset and duration. Epinephrine is contraindicated in areas where vasoconstriction could jeopardize the local circulation. This is not a problem with caudal injection.

Caudal morphine, 0.05–0.1 mg/kg, has a longer duration of analgesia than plain bupivacaine,[15] but a potentially increased incidence of nausea and vomiting, pruritus, sedation, and the possibility of delayed apnea. Fentanyl has similar adverse effects, with less risk of delayed apnea and little advantage in duration of action.[16] Whether the possible advantages of caudal morphine outweigh the disadvantages is controversial.[17]

Ketamine has been used caudally, has a number of theoretical advantages, but does not yet have an established place. Similarly, clonidine can provide analgesia by the caudal route,[17] but sedation is significantly increased. It may have a place for inpatients.

COMPLICATIONS

Failure of caudal block is uncommon with good technique and patient selection. Careful needle placement with confirmation of little resistance to injection, negative aspiration, and no visible swelling should prevent and detect subperiosteal, intraosseous or subcutaneous injections. Anatomical variants making detection of landmarks difficult or impossible are a common cause of failed block. Commencement of surgery shortly after the block is placed may result in inadequate onset time and reflex tachycardia, increased depth of respiration, or movement in response to surgery. In the recovery phase, young children may often be upset for reasons other than pain (for example, thirst, disorientation, or parental separation), making early postoperative assessment of the block difficult. Minimal intraoperative requirements for inhaled agents may be an excellent indicator of a successful block.

Overdose of local anesthetic drugs can be avoided by checking the dose per kilogram of drug used. This is especially important when a formula for volume required is used, as too high a concentration may be given. The maximum dose for bupivacaine infusions is 0.4 mg/kg per hour in children and 0.25 mg/kg per hour in neonates.[18] Separating local anesthetic agents from other drugs and not drawing up the local anesthetic solution until it is to be injected will minimize the risk of syringe swap and injection of the wrong drug.

'Bloody tap' is common. The incidence is lower with short bevel needles,[2] but some anesthesiologists prefer the feel of standard hypodermic needles for this block. Significant compressive hematoma also seems to be unreported in children after caudal injection.

Intravascular injection of local anesthetic solution is a rare but serious complication which may produce seizures and cardiac arrest. Meticulous attention to the possibility of intravascular injection, with repeated checks and slow injection, is important. The role of epinephrine or atropine as a marker is controversial. Needle insertion, even under general anesthesia, may provoke a tachycardia, masking the effects of intravenous epinephrine or atropine. Conversely, general anesthesia may blunt the response to epinephrine. Aspiration is not a completely reliable test. Disconnection of the syringe from the needle may reveal passive efflux of blood even when aspiration is negative. Having confirmed the absence of cerebrospinal fluid by aspiration and observation of the open needle hub prior to injection, momentary back-flow of clear local anesthetic solution on disconnection of the syringe immediately after a small (0.5–1 ml) rapid bolus injection of local anesthetic (which briefly raises the epidural pressure) provides definite confirmation that the needle is not intravascular. This procedure along with aspiration can be repeated several times during the injection to confirm that the needle has not entered a blood vessel. Disconnection raises a theoretical increased risk of bacterial contamination but this is unlikely with good aseptic technique.

Air embolus has recently been recognized as a complication of pediatric epidural injection.[19] Epidural air may be a cause of incomplete block. It is now recommended that air injection should be avoided.

Dural puncture occurs approximately once per 2500 pediatric caudal injections. It is more likely if the posterior sacrum is bifid more cephalad than usual (a relative contraindication to caudal injection if detected by palpation), and if a needle is threaded cranially up the caudal canal. Dural puncture headache is rare in small children and the main risk is inadvertent (and poorly managed) high or total spinal anesthesia.

Leg weakness is common with higher concentrations and volumes of local anesthetic solution. Moderate delay in postoperative micturition is common after caudal anesthesia, but established retention of urine is rare with a single injection. Perioperative incontinence may occur, especially if intraabdominal pressure is increased. Hypotension due to sympathetic block is rare in children after caudal anesthesia. It may occur with high blocks, relative hypovolemia, and in older children. Upper limb vasoconstriction compensates for the cardiovascular and thermoregulatory consequences of lower limb vasodilatation due to sympathetic blockade.[20] For sympathetic block to occur, the local anesthetic agent must reach the thoracolumbar sympathetic spinal outflow which ends about L1 or L2.

Infection has not been reported after single shot caudal injection in children, but has occurred after caudal catheter use for postoperative analgesia. Caudal catheter techniques are a standard form of postoperative analgesia in many centers.[21] Some centers prefer to use low lumbar or sacral intervertebral catheters for postoperative sacral blockade and direct placement of lumbar or thoracic epidural catheters as required, avoiding long caudal catheters. To minimize infection, whichever method is used, insertion must utilize meticulous sterile technique, the dressing should protect the site from contamination, the site should be inspected daily for signs of inflammation, and most catheters should be removed by the third day.

Ward complications may occur owing to failure to appreciate the presence of a caudal block, its effects and likely duration. Poor communication may leave ward staff unaware of the presence of a caudal block and concerned that the sensory and motor dysfunction is due to spinal pathology rather than local anesthesia. For operations where pain will be significant when the caudal blockade wears off, a plan for pain control at that time must be in place. Often prophylactic analgesia, especially acetaminophen (paracetamol), could be started in anticipation of the block receding, or intravenous access maintained to allow rapid commencement of an opioid infusion if required. The parents should also be aware of the expected effects, duration, and management of caudal blockade, especially for day patients. Ward staff (and parents) should be encouraged to obtain early anesthetic consultation if they believe the child is suffering an unexpected complication of caudal analgesia.

REFERENCES

1. Bosenberg AT, Bland BAR, Schulte-Steinberg O, Downing JW 1988 Thoracic epidural anesthesia via the caudal route in infants. Anesthesiology 69:267
2 Dalens B, Hasnaoui A 1989 Caudal anaesthesia in pediatric surgery: success rate and adverse effects in 750 consecutive patients. Anesthesia and Analgesia 68:83
3. Busoni P, Sarti A 1987 Sacral intervertebral epidural block. Anesthesiology 67:993
4. Gunter JB, Watcha MF, Forestner JE et al 1991 Caudal epidural anesthesia in conscious premature and high-risk infants. Journal of Pediatric Surgery 26:9–14
5. Takasaki M 1984 Blood concentrations of lidocaine, mepivacaine and bupivacaine during caudal analgesia in children. Acta Anesthesiologica Scandinavica 28:211
6. Rothstein P, Arthur GR, Feldman HS, Kopf GS, Covino BG 1986 Bupivacaine for intercostal nerve blocks in children: blood concentrations and pharmacokinetics. Anesthesia and Analgesia 65:625
7. Busoni P, Andreuccetti T 1986 The spread of caudal analgesia in children: a mathematical model. Anesthesia and Intensive Care 14:140–144
8. Schulte-Steinberg O, Rahlfs VW 1977 Spread of extradural analgesia following caudal injection in children. A statistical study. British Journal of Anesthesia 49:1027–1034
9. Wolf AR, Valley RD, Fear DW, Lawrence RW, Lerman J 1988 Bupivacaine for caudal anesthesia for infants and children: the optimal effective concentration. Anesthesiology 69:102
10. Gunter JB, Dunn CM, Bennie JB, Pentecost DL, Bower RJ, Ternberg JL 1991 Optimum concentration of bupivacaine for combined caudal-general anesthesia in children. Anesthesiology 75:57
11. Spear RM 1991 Dose-response in infants receiving caudal anesthesia with bupivacaine. Paediatric Anaesthesia 1:47–52
12. Eyres RL, Bishop W, Oppenheim RC, Brown TCK 1983 Plasma bupivacaine concentrations in children during caudal epidural analgesia. Anesthesia and Intensive Care 11:20
13. Warner MA, Kunkal SE, Offord KO, Atchison SR, Dawson B 1987 The effects of age, epinephrine and operation site on duration of caudal anesthesia in pediatric patients. Anesthesia and Analgesia, 66:995
14. Jamali S, Monin S, Begon C, Dubousset AM, Ecoffey C 1994 Clonidine in pediatric caudal anesthesia. Anesthesia and Analgesia. 78:663–666
15. Wolf AR, Hughes D, Wade A, Mather SJ, Prys-Roberts C 1990 Postoperative analgesia after paediatric orchidopexy: evaluation of a bupivacaine–morphine mixture. British Journal of Anesthesia 64:430
16. Campbell FA, Yentis SM, Fear DW, Bissonnette B 1992 Analgesic efficacy and safety of a caudal bupivacaine–fentanyl mixture in children. Canadian Journal of Anesthesia 39:661–664. (erratum: Canadian Journal of Anesthesia 1993, 40:288)
17. Bosenberg AT 1993 Caudal epidural morphine in children – a need for caution: (letter). South African Medical Journal 83:367
18. McCloskey JJ, Haun SE 1992 Deshpande JK 1992 Bupivacaine toxicity secondary to continuous caudal epidural infusion in children. Anesthesia and Analgesia 75:287–290 (see also editorial, same issue)
19. Guinard JP, Borboen M 1993 Probable venous air embolism during caudal anesthesia in a child. Anesthesia and Analgesia 76:1134–1135 (see also editorial, same issue)
20. Payen D, Ecoffey C, Carli P, Dubousset AM 1987 Pulsed Doppler ascending aortic, carotid, brachial, and femoral artery blood flows during caudal anesthesia in infants. Anesthesiology 67:681–685
21. Gunter JB, Eng C 1992 Thoracic epidural anesthesia via the caudal approach in children. Anesthesiology 76:935–938

9 Nerve blocks for analgesia

Kester Brown

The advantage of individual nerve blocks is that sensory block can be achieved without the widespread autonomic and motor block which often results from major regional blocks. Nerve blocks after induction of anesthesia can reduce general anesthetic requirements during surgery and improve recovery.

In the operating room, local anesthetic blocks are normally used in conjunction with general anesthesia, but they can be performed in awake children with or without sedation, especially in older children. When performed under general anesthesia the procedure should be done before surgery to provide operative and postoperative analgesia. Accident and emergency departments often underutilize nerve blocks in conscious children. If the patient is not anesthetized, local anesthetic cream makes skin puncture painless and the injection should not cause discomfort if it is in the correct space and is not impinging on the nerve. Injection should not be made if there is resistance (see Ch. 20 for a discussion of techniques of local anesthesia in awake children, especially Table 20.2). Paresthesia or pain on injection from intraneural placement cannot be detected in anesthetized children.

Unless repeated blocks or a catheter for infusion of a local anesthetic agent are used, pain may develop as the block wears off. There should be a plan to introduce other analgesics (e.g. a loading dose of 25–30 mg/kg acetaminophen (paracetamol)) so that they are effective before the local anesthetic action wears off. The choice of drug will depend on the surgery and the amount of tissue damage. Simple analgesics such as acetaminophen can also be used as a supplement to relieve pain not covered by the block.

The simplest way of applying local anesthesia is topically or by infiltration. Infiltration of the wound can be performed by the surgeon. Examples of topical analgesia for surgical pain include the application of lidocaine (lignocaine) ointment to the penis following circumcision when other forms of analgesia are wearing off,[1] and spraying of the tonsillar fossae after tonsillectomy (Fig. 9.1). Infiltration local anesthesia (as with nerve blocks) done after induction of general anesthesia rather than at the end of surgery can minimize the amount of intraoperative general anesthetic agent required.

GENERAL CONSIDERATIONS

The use of nerve blocks requires a good understanding of the anatomy and the principles of locating depth so that the local anesthetic solution

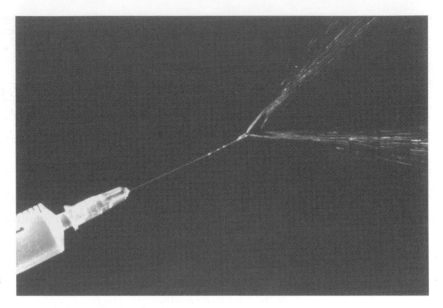

Fig. 9.1 A 21 gauge needle with the tip bent so that the fluid when injected sprays to cover the tonsil fossa evenly with local anesthetic solution (0.5–1ml bupivacaine 0.5% on each side)

can be deposited accurately around the nerve. The location of depth is assisted by:

- Using a short beveled needle so that a loss of resistance or 'pop' is felt easily as it is inserted gently through fascia or aponeurosis
- The fact that it is difficult to inject when light pressure is applied to the plunger of the syringe when the needle tip is in muscle or dense fibrous tissue, but becomes easy when the tip enters a potential space between layers. Nerves often traverse such spaces and are blocked by flooding the space with local anesthetic solution

Where the nerve is subcutaneous a single injection over the point where the nerve is most likely to lie can be spread by squeezing between two fingers rather than running the needle subcutaneously (Fig. 9.2).

Equipment

A short beveled block needle (22 gauge is commonly used in children) should be used, if available, for blocks where fascial layers need to be felt, and may be less likely to damage a nerve than sharper needles. In the simplest situation, nerve blocks can be performed with a syringe, needle, local anesthetic and antiseptic solution to cleanse the skin. More specialized equipment such as a nerve stimulator, prepacked kits and catheters are helpful when indicated.

An extension set attached between the syringe and needle can be used to help immobilize the needle in the position for injection. Alternatively, gripping the needle with a hand resting on the patient while injecting with the other can successfully immobilize the needle. Preventing movement of the needle tip once the space is identified is important in small children where the spaces containing nerves are very shallow.

Nerve stimulators which deliver a short pulse (40–100 microseconds) with a low maximum current (less than 3 mA) can be used to confirm the location

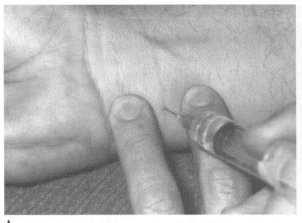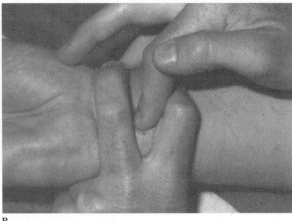

A   B

Fig. 9.2 (A,B) The local anesthetic agent injected near the expected site of a subcutaneous nerve at the wrist or ankle can be spread laterally and medially with pressure using two fingers to prevent proximal and distal spread

of a nerve.[2] A Teflon-coated needle, completely insulated except for the tip, aids accurate localization of nerves and protects against direct muscle stimulation. The needle tip needs to be near the nerve to obtain a response. Some needles have tubing attached to make injection with an immobile needle easier. The current used in small children should be low and gradually increased until an adequate response is achieved. Placement very close to the nerve is confirmed by stimulation using a low current (e.g. 0.5 mA) with cessation of response when a small volume (0.3 ml) is injected.

Consultation

It is advisable to discuss the use of nerve blocks beforehand with the surgeon to ensure there are no surgical contraindications and to confirm that the operative site will be covered by the nerves to be blocked. The parents, and if appropriate the child, should be told about planned use of blocks. Care of the numb limb should be mentioned and older children warned of abnormal sensation. Any concerns can be discussed at that time.

Complications

Nerve damage

Trauma or injection into a nerve causing neuropraxia or neuralgia very occasionally occurs after a nerve block and the patient complains of continuing discomfort. The anesthesiologist should be informed. Because the anesthetized child cannot complain of paresthesia or pain, it is important that the anesthesiologist ensures that the bevel of the needle is parallel to and not across the nerve and *only injects when it is easy to do so* in order to avoid damage. If there is significant resistance the needle tip is probably not in the correct position and may be in the nerve.

Ischemia

Pain may be an indication that a plaster is too tight when applied following limb surgery, that there is compartment compression, or that pressure necrosis is developing. If a nerve block is used this warning is lost. Usually the anesthesiologist should discuss the proposed use of blocks with the surgeon beforehand so that particular care can be taken when applying plaster, and the ward staff must know so that they can watch for other signs of ischemia such as poor perfusion of toes and fingers. Ischemia is also a hazard when epinephrine (adrenaline) is used in areas supplied by end arteries. It must *never* be used for penile or digital blocks.

Choice and dose of local anesthetic agent

When postoperative analgesia is desired a long-acting drug such as bupivacaine is most appropriate. Some prolongation of action may be achieved by adding epinephrine 1:200 000–1:400 000 or by using infusion via catheters. The concentration for surgical analgesia is 0.25%, although up to 0.5% is used if motor block is necessary. A concentration of 0.125% is usually adequate for postoperative infusions. If lidocaine is the only drug available it can be used, but its action is too short to provide prolonged postoperative analgesia unless an infusion is used.

The dose of local anesthetic drug should be limited. Usually 3 mg/kg bupivacaine, 5 mg/kg lidocaine, or 7 mg/kg lidocaine with epinephrine are safe. Blood levels with these doses will not usually reach toxic levels unless the drugs are injected intravascularly, when smaller doses may cause toxicity – convulsions, bradycardia, and decreased cardiac output. The central nervous system signs may be masked by general anesthesia although they will occur with higher blood levels.

Toxicity of local anesthetic drugs

The uptake of local anesthetic drugs into the blood and their toxicity depends on the vascular supply of the area, the dose, the concentration, and the child's age. Most peripheral nerves are in less vascular areas than, for example, the epidural space. Quoted safe doses[3] are fairly conservative, and 3 mg/kg[4] and even 4 mg/kg[5] of bupivacaine have been used epidurally. Serious toxic reactions such as convulsions or myocardial depression can occur with intravascular injection.[6] These may result from doses much below the safe recommended dose. Peak blood levels and therefore toxicity vary with the site of injection.[7] It is important to aspirate before injecting to ensure that the needle is not in a blood vessel. Occasionally intravascular injection can occur when no blood is aspirated. Facilities and staff for cardiopulmonary resuscitation should be immediately available. If a serious reaction occurs the patient must immediately be ventilated with oxygen.

SPECIFIC BLOCKS

The techniques for nerve blocks are covered in detail in other books[8,9] but a few commonly used in children are described here with details of techniques that have proved useful in increasing the reliability of the block. Nerve blocks of the face and distal part of the limbs are particularly useful in conscious older children with lacerations or fractures which are suitable for repair or reduction in the emergency department. The management of these patients as well as details of topical, infiltration, and intravenous regional anesthesia are described in Chapter 20. Local anesthetic blockade should give profound analgesia if correctly placed and an adequate concentration is used.

Ilioinguinal and iliohypogastric nerve block

Ilioinguinal and iliohypogastric nerve blocks are used for inguinal hernia and hydrocele repairs, and inguinal incisions for varicocele surgery and orchidopexy. Block of the ilioinguinal and iliohypogastric nerves alone, deep to the external oblique aponeurosis, provides cutaneous anesthesia but misses the deeper structures. This block can either be performed under direct vision during surgery or performed percutaneously by the anesthesiologist. More extensive blockade is provided by a field block involving a deeper injection to cover the inguinal canal, while the cutaneous block can be provided by direct infiltration.

The following description is for preoperative percutaneous insertion which provides analgesia throughout surgery. A short beveled needle is inserted about 1 cm medial to the anterior superior iliac spine in a small child (less in a baby and up to 2 cm in an older child) (Fig. 9.3). The needle is advanced gently until a resistance is felt – there is a loss of resistance or a 'pop' as the needle passes through the external oblique aponeurosis. At this point 0.25 ml/kg of 0.25% bupivacaine can be injected. The needle is then advanced slowly with pressure on the plunger of the syringe. It is difficult to inject while passing through the internal oblique muscle. When the space between it and the transversus abdominis muscle is reached, injection becomes easy. A volume of 0.25 ml/kg of local anesthetic solution instilled in this layer will pass down around the neck of the hernia sac providing analgesia for that part of the operation (Fig. 9.4). Massaging in the direction desired will help the spread of the local anesthetic solution. With good surgical cooperation, the success of the block can be improved by running a

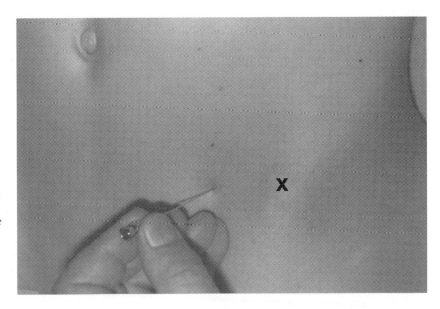

Fig. 9.3 The needle is inserted 1–2 cm medial to the anterior superior iliac spine (marked X) depending on the size of the child. Note the hand is resting on the abdominal wall so that the needle tip is held steady when the relevant spaces are located

Fig. 9.4 The layers through which the needle is inserted in an ilioinguinal and iliohypogastric nerve block. Half the volume (0.25 ml/kg) is injected between the external and internal oblique muscles to block the nerves. The needle is then advanced further with pressure on the plunger; injection becomes easy when the space between the internal oblique and transversus muscles is reached. This space contains the neck of the hernia sac medially (ASIS, anterior superior iliac spine; Ext. Obl. ap. external oblique aponewosis; Int. Obl. m., internal oblique muscle)

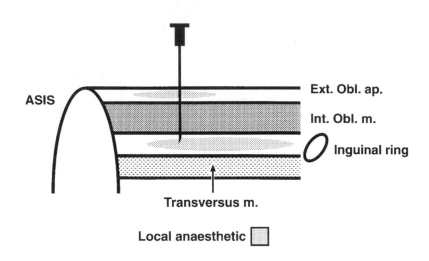

subcutaneous weal of local anesthetic from the initial injection site along the proposed line of the incision before withdrawing the block needle.

The deeper injection may occasionally produce femoral nerve block. This block can be used in neonates, but requires gentleness and sensitivity to feel the thin layers. If a short beveled needle is not available the external oblique aponeurosis can be located with an ordinary needle by moving it gently up and down in a cephalocaudal plane until a rough, irregular sensation like dragging a needle over a palm leaf is felt. These are the fibers of the external oblique aponeurosis which can then be penetrated. Another trick is to pass the needle at an angle so that a greater thickness of aponeurosis has to be penetrated.

Penile block

There are several techniques for providing analgesia for circumcision, including a ring block around the distal penis or injection into the triangular space bounded by the symphysis pubis, corpus cavernosum and fascia (Fig. 9.5). The fascia divides in the midline to form the suspensory ligament of the penis which then divides around the penis. The dorsal nerves and vessels lie deep to this (Fig. 9.6). On either side of the suspensory ligament there are potential spaces which open up on injection of fluid (Fig. 9.7). A midline injection usually only fills one side. The recommended technique is to inject local anesthetic solution bilaterally to fill these spaces. As there are ventral branches arising posteriorly which supply the area around the frenulum, it is important to inject a large enough volume of the solution (1 ml plus 0.1 ml/kg on each side) to pass posteriorly to block these branches. *Never* use epinephrine.

The technique is to put the skin and fascia on stretch by pushing the penis downwards. The needle is inserted into the space first angled to one side and then the other. If a short beveled needle is used a 'pop' may be felt as the fascia is penetrated. The needle is advanced until it is easy to inject – this is when the needle tip is in the potential space from which the

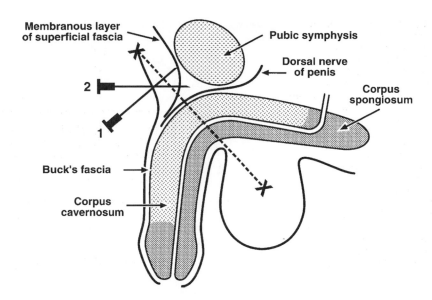

Fig. 9.5 Dorsal nerve of penis block. Lateral view demonstrating the space bounded by the symphysis pubis, corpora cavernosa and fascia where the local anesthetic solution is deposited. The ventral branch is also blocked when a sufficient volume (1 ml plus 0.1 ml/kg on each side) is injected to spread posteriorly to fill the space

local anesthetic agent readily diffuses to the nerves. Injection into the deep space containing the nerves is dangerous because puncture of a blood vessel may result in a hematoma, vascular compression, and ischemia of parts of the penis. Always aspirate before injection.

Intercostal block

The increase in use of epidural analgesia has resulted in intercostal block being less commonly used. It is still an easy block which can be performed quickly, and if attempted carefully and gently can be used even in neonates. Sometimes the surgeon injects the intercostal space under direct vision when the chest is open, but this means that the local anesthetic agent is not acting during the opening incision, which is the most painful

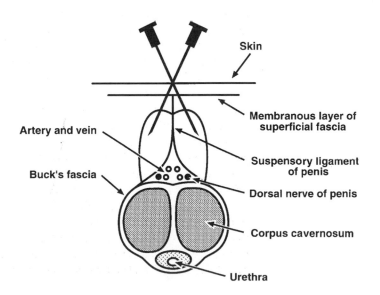

Fig. 9.6 Dorsal nerve of penis block. A cross-section of the space shown in Fig. 9.4 showing how the suspensory ligament of the penis divides the space. Local anesthetic solution injected on either side into a pear-shaped potential space will diffuse into the space where the nerves and vessels lie

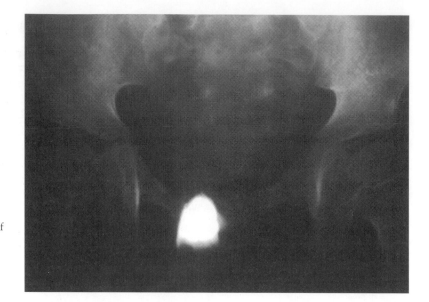

Fig. 9.7 Radiograph demonstrating dye in one of the spaces lateral to the suspensory ligament of the penis where the local anesthetic drug should be injected

period of surgery. Intercostal blocks are also useful in the management of fractured ribs and in the treatment of localized pain in the region.

The block can be performed, usually after the induction of anesthesia, either as a series of injections or by injecting a larger volume at one space. The latter technique depends on medial spread of the local anesthetic solution until it reaches the paravertebral region where it can spread to the spaces above and below, because in this area the parietal pleura and fascia are only loosely attached to the ribs allowing free flow of fluid. The volume needed to reach this area will be less if the needle is inserted just lateral to the paravertebral muscles rather than further laterally at the angle of the rib (Fig. 9.8).

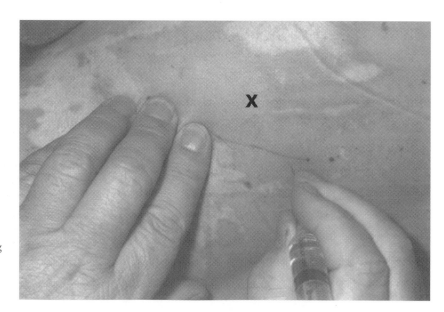

Fig. 9.8 Intercostal block. The patient is lying on their right side in the photograph. The needle is inserted just lateral to the paravertebral muscles. The left hand fingers are delineating the ribs. The right hand is resting on the back, controlling the needle which is inserted just below the rib. 'X' marks the angle of the rib

The technique is to count the ribs from below to locate the space or spaces to be blocked. The hand holding the needle is positioned on the chest wall so that the relationship of the needle to the chest wall is controlled and the lung is not accidentally punctured by sudden movement or coughing. The needle is inserted directly over the rib until it is contacted, then gradually moved down the rib until it reaches the lower border and advances through the external intercostal muscle. This can be felt, even in a neonate, as a rough, grating sensation as the needle penetrates the fibers. The needle is advanced until injection is easy, after ensuring that the tip is not in a vessel. Despite diagrams showing the vessels and nerves lying behind the groove on the lower edge of the rib this is not usually the case – they can be lying in the middle of the space, where they can be punctured by the needle.

Only small volumes of local anesthetic solution are needed to block each nerve individually, while larger volumes are needed if one injection is used to block several spaces because the local anesthetic solution must fill the space and then traverse up and down – it may require 5 ml in an infant and up to 20 ml in an adolescent (0.3–0.5 ml/kg of 0.25% bupivacaine) (Fig. 9.8). If epinephrine is added the duration of the block is prolonged.

If the proposed incision crosses the midline, a limited number of bilateral intercostal blocks can be used. This is safer in infants because their ribs are more horizontal than in older patients and their intercostal muscles thus play a less important role in respiration compared with the diaphragm.

Intercostal blocks are often done as a single injection with a long-acting local anesthetic agent. If necessary, this can be repeated, or a catheter technique can be used in older children, but often one injection will provide analgesia for up to 18 hours.

The technique can be used for thoracic or abdominal procedures – a right 11th space block is useful for postoperative analgesia following appendicectomy.

Femoral nerve block

Femoral nerve block is useful in the management of fractured shaft of femur, incisions over its cutaneous distribution, and cropping of split skin for grafting. The femoral nerve can be located just lateral to the femoral artery below the inguinal ligament. As it lies in a canal deep to fascia lata and fascia iliaca, two 'pops' or losses of resistance are usually felt as these are penetrated with a short beveled needle (Fig. 9.9). There is almost no resistance to injection if the needle is in the correct location. If not, it may be that the fascial layers are fused, and the needle is in the muscle deep to the canal or in the nerve. Withdrawal of the needle until injection is easy will usually achieve successful block. Injection of 0.3 ml/kg of 0.25 to 0.5% bupivacaine will produce a good femoral nerve block. If a larger volume is used, such as 0.7 ml/kg of 0.25% bupivacaine, a three-in-one block including lateral cutaneous nerve of thigh and obturator nerve may result. Prolonged analgesia can be maintained by insertion of a catheter into the canal carrying the femoral nerve and infusing local anesthetic solution.

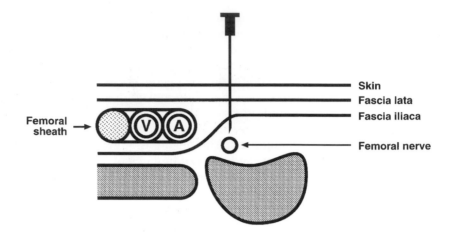

Fig. 9.9 Femoral nerve block showing the fascial layers that must be penetrated to find the canal with the femoral nerve

Sciatic nerve block

The sciatic nerve can be blocked to provide analgesia in the posterior lower leg and foot and to relieve pain in fractured tibia or fibula. It can be blocked at several sites, but in the posterior midthigh where it lies deep to the biceps femoris muscle it is easily accessible (Fig. 9.10). A needle inserted perpendicularly through the skin into the muscle is then advanced with pressure on the plunger of the syringe until injection is easy. This loss of resistance is felt as the needle emerges from the muscle into the space containing the sciatic nerve. The instillation of local anesthetic in this space will bathe the nerve. Accurate location of the nerve can be confirmed by a nerve stimulator.

Blocks at the ankle

The nerve supply to the foot and ankle is shown in Figures 9.11–9.14.

Posterior tibial nerve block produces anesthesia of the sole of the foot except posteriorly (see opposite). The posterior tibial nerve divides to form

Fig. 9.10 The landmarks for the midthigh sciatic nerve block (McKenzie approach). Inject at the point marked 'x', where the biceps femoris (attached to the ischial tuberosity and the head of the fibula) crosses the sciatic nerve (passing from the midpoint of the line from ischial tuberosity and greater trochanter and the apex of the popliteal fossa). The injection site is just proximal to the apex of the popliteal fossa, in the midline. The injection is made deep to the long head of biceps femoris (see text)

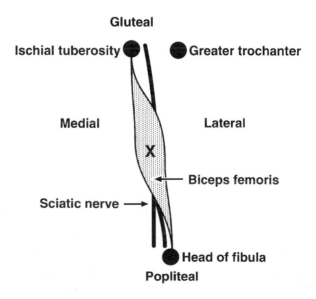

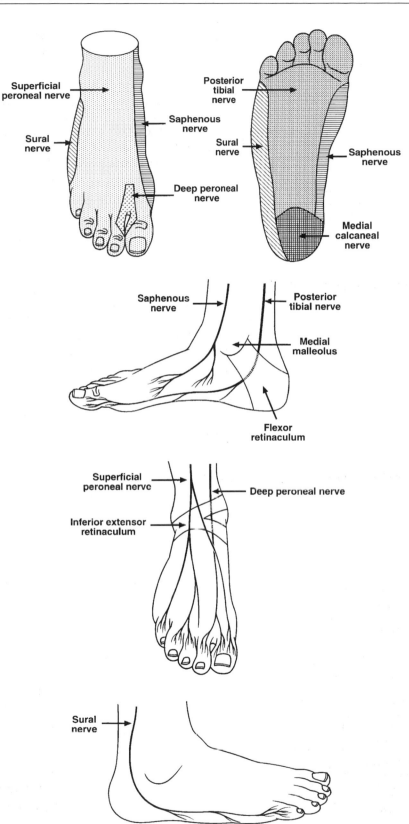

Fig. 9.11   Distribution of the cutaneous nerve supply of the foot. The boundaries of these areas of distribution vary. The saphenous nerve distribution may include the medial aspect of the great (first) toe and the sural nerve the lateral aspect of the little (fifth) toe

Fig. 9.12   Medial view of ankle and foot. Note that the posterior tibial nerve accompanies the artery and is deep to the retinaculum

Fig. 9.13   Dorsum of foot and anterior aspect of ankle. Note that the deep peroneal nerve accompanies the dorsalis pedis artery and is deep to the retinaculum

Fig. 9.14   Lateral view of the foot and ankle showing the course of the sural nerve which is subcutaneous

the medial and lateral plantar nerves. The nerve is blocked by injecting 2–3 ml of local anesthetic solution posterior to the posterior tibial artery as it passes deep to the flexor retinaculum between the medial malleolus and the calcaneum. Injection superficial to this tough fascial layer will not block the nerve. The deep peroneal nerve is also deep to fascia and can be blocked deep to the extensor retinaculum, lateral to the dorsalis pedis artery. It supplies the skin of the first web space. Palpating the artery and injecting deep to the fascia are the keys to both these blocks.

The other nerves at the ankle are subcutaneous. The saphenous nerve lies anterolateral to the medial malleolus. It supplies the medial aspect of the foot. The superficial peroneal nerve runs anteromedial to the lateral malleolus and supplies most of the skin of the dorsum of the foot. The sural nerve lies halfway between the lateral malleolus and the calcaneum, supplying the lateral aspect of the foot. The medial calcaneal branches of the posterior tibial nerve arise medially above the ankle and supply the posterior heel. Transverse subcutaneous injections of local anesthetic solution in these regions will block these nerves.

As the boundaries of the distribution of these nerves are variable and there is overlap of supply from contiguous nerves, it is often wise to block the nerves on either side of the surgical field as well as those directly involved. Infiltration of the weight-bearing areas of the plantar surface of the foot is often very painful owing to the high pressure that local anesthetic injection produces in the fibrous compartments of the sole of the foot. Nerve blocks at the ankle can produce anesthesia of these areas with less pain on injection.

Brachial plexus block

Brachial plexus blocks can be used in children. The axillary approach is most commonly used. The arm is abducted, the brachial artery palpated, and the needle is inserted beside it. A 'pop' may be felt when the sheath carrying the plexus is penetrated. If a large volume (0.3–0.5 ml/kg 0.25% bupivacaine) of local anesthetic solution relative to the patient's size is injected, it will bathe the plexus.

Digital nerve block

There are two methods of performing a digital nerve block.

The first method involves blocking each digital nerve at the level of the proximal phalanx (Fig. 9.15). Insert the needle into the side of the digit at the lateral or medial aspect of the ventral surface at a 45 degree angle to the vertical with the palm up until the periosteum is hit, and then inject. Then rotate the needle to vertical and inject along the side of the finger to at least three-quarters of the digit depth. Remove the needle and repeat on other side of finger. *Note:* for the index and little fingers a half-ring weal of lidocaine along the radial and ulnar sides of each finger is needed to achieve adequate anesthesia.

The second method involves blocking the nerve at the level of the metacarpophalangeal joint. This may be less painful. Insert the needle between the fingers at the interdigital fold in line with the web space. Insert to a depth of 1–2 cm (i.e. the tip is at the level of the metacarpophalangeal joint) and inject 1–2ml of local anesthetic solution.

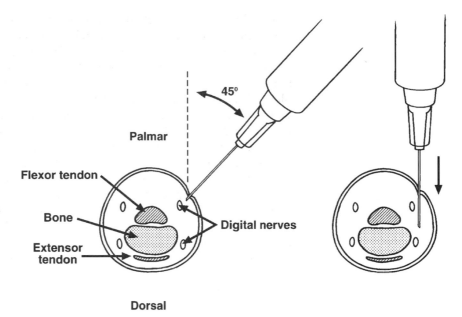

Fig. 9.15 Digital nerve block – cross-section of the proximal first phalanx. After penetration of the skin and advancement towards the bone, the needle is turned in an anteroposterior direction and local anesthetic solution injected in that line

Ulnar nerve block

The ulnar nerve runs deep and lateral to the flexor-carpi ulnaris muscle at the level of the wrist joint. An ulnar nerve block produces anesthesia of the medial third of the palm, the little finger and metacarpal, and the medial side of the ring finger (palmar aspect).

There are two methods (Fig. 9.16):

- Inject 2–3 ml of local anesthetic solution from the medial side of the wrist under flexor-carpi ulnaris and 1–2 cm proximal to the wrist skin crease, to a depth of 1–2 cm
- Inject 2–3 ml of local anesthetic solution directly medial to flexor-carpi ulnaris and perpendicular to the wrist, to a depth of 0.5 cm

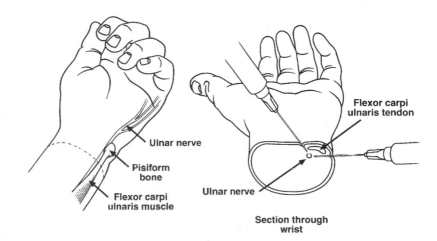

Fig. 9.16 Ulnar nerve block. Course of the ulnar nerve in relation to the flexor carpi ulnaris muscle and tendon. The nerve may be approached from anteriorly, lateral to the tendon of flexor carpi ulnaris, or medially, passing the needle posterior to the tendon of flexor carpi ulnaris

Median nerve block

Median nerve block (Fig. 9.17) at the wrist produces anesthesia of the whole tip and anterior half of the thumb, index and middle fingers, lateral half of the ring finger, and lateral aspect of palm. In some patients the recurrent nerve branches off before the flexor retinaculum, so distal block-ade will not cover the palm, unless a more superficial injection is also made. The injection is made lateral to palmaris longus at a depth of 0.5 cm, deep to the retinaculum, with 2–3 ml of local anesthetic solution. An alternative method to ensure the correct depth and minimize the risk of nerve injury is to pass the needle from laterally under the palmaris longus tendon. In children with an absent palmaris longus tendon the injection is made medial to flexor carpi radialis. In adults this block has a significant incidence of residual paresthesia, and alternatives are preferred.

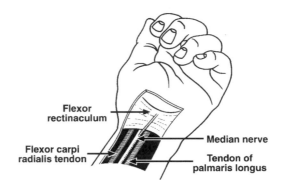

Fig. 9.17 Median nerve block. The palmaris longus tendon often overlies the median nerve. If the palmaris longus is absent, injection can be made medial to the tendon of flexor carpi radialis

Infraorbital nerve block

Infraorbital nerve block (Figs 9.18–9.20) produces anesthesia of the upper lip and cheek from the midline and tip of the nose. The injection is made superficial to the infraorbital foramen which can be palpated in the same plane as the pupil below the infraorbital rim. The intraoral approach is less painful. After topical anesthesia of the mucobuccal junction, posterior to the canine tooth, the needle is passed in the direction of the infraorbital foramen, and 1–2 ml of local anesthetic solution injected. Injection in the infraorbital canal can damage the nerve.

Mental nerve block

Mental nerve block (Figs 9.18–9.20) produces anesthesia of the lower lip and jaw lateral to the midline. The mental nerve exits the mandible at the level of the premolar through the mental foramen, which is palpable in the same sagittal plane as the supraorbital and infraorbital foramina. As with the infraorbital block, an intraoral approach can be used via the mucobuccal junction just above this point, taking care to inject 1–2 ml of local anesthetic solution superficial to the foramen.

Supraorbital nerve block

Supraorbital nerve block (Figs 9.18, 9.19) produces anesthesia of the fore-head and scalp. With combined block of the supratrochlear nerve (see below) this will extend from the midline and up to the vertex. The injection is made superficial to the supraorbital foramen which can be palpat-ed in the same plane as the pupil above the supraorbital rim. The needle

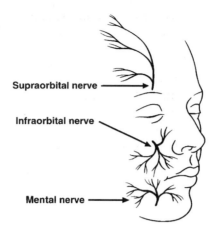

Fig. 9.18   Distribution of the supraorbital, infraorbital, and mental nerves

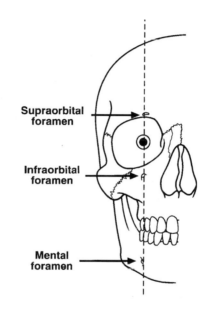

Fig. 9.19   In adults and older children, the supraorbital, infraorbital, and mental foramina are in the same sagittal plane as the pupil. Care must be taken to avoid injecting local anesthetic solution in a foramen

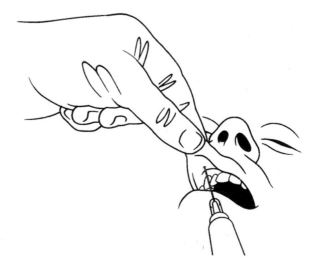

Fig. 9.20   The intraoral approach to infraorbital nerve block. A similar approach in the mucobuccal junction of the lower jaw can be used for mental nerve block

is passed perpendicularly to the path of the nerve above the supraorbital foramen, and 1–2 ml of local anesthetic solution injected. Injection in the supraorbital canal can damage the nerve. The supratrochlear nerve runs just medial to the supraorbital nerve and supplies a portion of the skin of the forehead, eyelid and eyebrow medially and above the orbit. It may be blocked by infiltrating medially to the supraorbital nerve.

Summary

Nerve blocks are useful for the provision of analgesia during and following many types of surgery in children. Some, such as femoral or sciatic blocks, are useful to provide analgesia during transportation, radiography and treatment of limb fractures. It is important to understand the anatomy when performing nerve blocks if reliable results are to be achieved. Appropriate reference books should be consulted for any blocks not fully described in this chapter.

REFERENCES

1   Tritrakarn T, Pirayavaraporn S, Lertakyamanee J 1987 Topical analgesia for relief of post-circumcision pain. Anesthesiology 67:395
2. Deleur MM 1990 Equipment. In: Saint-Maurice C, Schulte-Steinberg O (eds) Regional anaesthesia for children. Mediglobe, Fribourg, pp 68–75
3. Covino B 1988 Clinical pharmacology of local anesthetic agents. In: Cousins MJ, Bridenbaugh PO, (eds) Neural blockade, 2nd edn. JB Lippincott, Philadelphia, p 112
4. Eyres RL, Hastings C, Brown TCK, Oppenheim RC 1986 Plasma bupivacaine concentrations following lumbar epidural anaesthesia in children. Anaesthesia and Intensive Care 14:131
5. Melman E, Arenas JA, Tandazo WE 1985 Caudal anaesthesia for paediatric surgery. An easy and safe method for calculating dose requirements. Anesthesiology 63:A463
6. Eyres RL, Hastings C, Brown TCK 1983 Plasma level of bupivacaine during convulsions. Anaesthesia and Intensive Care 11:385
7. Brown TCK, Fisk GC 1990 Anaesthesia for children, 2nd edn. Blackwell, Oxford, p 45
8. Cousins MJ, Bridenbaugh PO 1988 Neural blockade, 2nd edn. JB Lippincott, Philadelphia, ch 21
9. Brown TCK, Fisk GC 1990 Anaesthesia for children, 2nd edn. Blackwell, Oxford, ch 22

10 Pain assessment

Ian McKenzie

INTRODUCTION

In any child known to have a potentially painful condition, pain assessment should be routine and repeated. If the pain assessment indicates unacceptable pain is present, the further assessment of that pain should be a diagnostic exercise. Could the pain reasonably be caused by the patient's known condition? Is that condition being properly treated? If this pain is not typical of the patient's known condition, what is the new cause and how should that be treated? What analgesic methods have been tried so far, and how effective were they? Other causes of distress that may worsen the pain experience, such as fear, anxiety, cold, hunger and thirst, should be assessed and addressed. Pain assessment is part of pain management, which is more than the application of increasingly potent analgesics.

The assessment of pain will not improve the management of pain unless the assessment produces appropriate action. Inadequate pain relief should not only be charted, but treated. If the currently prescribed treatment is ineffective, a clear referral path should be in place so that consultation and further assessment and treatment can be instituted as soon as an unsatisfactory pain management plan is detected.

PAIN ASSESSMENT IN CHILDREN

The fact that pain is a subjective experience means that anybody with problems communicating will have more difficulty conveying not only that they are in pain but also the site, nature, and severity of the pain. Although a wide variety of disorders of communication may occur at any age, in pediatrics the developmentally appropriate difficulty with communication of normal infants and young children is the commonest cause of difficulties with pain assessment.

There are many methods that may be used to help the clinician in arriving at an assessment, either by assisting the patient's expression such as visual analog scales (VAS), 'face' scales (e.g. Wong-Baker or Bieri[1]) (Fig. 10.1) or by formally scoring various observable clinical factors such as heart and respiratory rates, mobility, demeanor and patient report, for example the All India Institute of Medical Science pain/discomfort scale.[2] In small children, the family may assist assessment by describing the

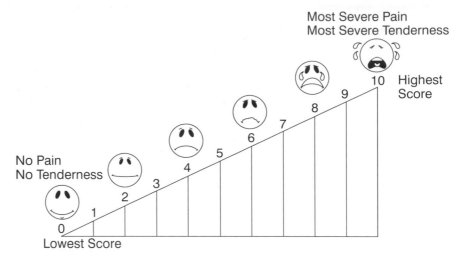

Fig. 10.1 A visual analog scale for pain, incorporating a 'faces' scale

patient's previous behavior in response to pain, or perhaps distinguish distress due to pain from distress due to other causes.

To produce a VAS the patient is asked to mark where the current pain would lie on a 10 cm line with one end representing 'no pain', the other 'the worst pain you have experienced'. This wording is of some importance, because saying the 'pain' end represents 'the worst pain you can imagine' can evoke nightmarish thoughts of mutilation and torture that may distress some children. The score is the distance from the 'no pain' end to the patient's mark. Few children under 7 years old will be able to grasp the concept of the VAS. The score should not be taken at face value. Interpretation must take into account the patient's whole clinical state. An apparently unsatisfactory high score may represent an improvement on a previous score, or be an expression of the patient's anger with staff or circumstances rather than a 'pure' measure of pain. Each patient will tend to have different ideas about what score represents a pain that is reasonably tolerable.

The 'faces' pain scale is a series of simple line drawings of faces expressing various degrees of pain from none to extreme (Fig. 10.1). Children as young as 4 years old can grasp the concept of selecting the face that best represents their current pain. Some modifications align these faces beside a VAS style line which can be marked by the patient. Ideally, the faces scale should be validated, specific, use a 'no pain' face rather than a happy face at one end of the scale, and consecutive faces should represent equal intervals across the full spectrum of pain severity.[1]

Although appearing more scientific, these methods have advantages and disadvantages, and are not inherently better than a clinical assessment by an experienced carer with a personal relationship with the patient (and the patient's family). Clinically, the goal of a quantitative assessment of pain need only be to categorize the pain as absent, mild, moderate, or severe. Even if one of these scoring systems is being used, clinical management will usually be based on (sometimes unconsciously) converting that score to a simple description of the pain as absent, mild, moderate, or severe. The charting, preferably with other routine observations, of whatever pain assessment is used is important for continuity of patient care and overall assessment.

Pain assessment in children too young to describe their pain is a difficult problem. The nonspecific nature of their reaction to pain means that the distress must be viewed in context and a clinical management plan produced. The connection between crying after a needle-stick procedure and the procedure itself is clinically obvious. An infant with a source of acute pain (e.g. postoperative pain) that will take days to resolve is likely to cry for many reasons other than pain during that time, yet each episode of crying raises the possibility of unsatisfactory pain management. Various 'objective pain scores' (e.g. the AIIMS pain/discomfort scale)[2] have been suggested, usually involving summation of points allocated for various observable behaviors and physiological measurements (such as pulse rate). These provide some standardization and guidance about what to look for when assessing a child. However, as there is no 'gold standard' the scores cannot be validated in infants, they usually score sedation as analgesia, and there is no evidence that they are better than an experienced observer (with full knowledge of the patient's clinical condition) rating the pain as absent, mild, moderate, or severe.

A second difficult problem in assessing pain in young children is diagnosing the child who withdraws in response to pain. These children will commonly look pale (sympathetic activity) and show no interest in their surroundings. This appearance may resemble that of children with serious disorders (e.g. hypoxia or hypotension) or children who are stressed and withdrawn owing to the hospital environment or sleep deprivation. Hospital staff need to notice these children and diagnose them, though the temptation is to ignore the quiet child. Similarly, excessive sedation produces a quiet child who is at risk of serious complications, and it should not be assumed that a quiet child is a happy, healthy child.

Giving analgesics to a baby who is crying because of hunger seems inappropriate (if the child can be fed), yet if feeding and general comforting settles a child in pain, may this be better than administering analgesics with potential side-effects? The management of a small child thought to be in pain is unlikely to be based on a totally scientific rationale, and the art of clinical practice is gaining a knowledge of the patient, the illness, and possible management options, leading to the 'best guess' implementation of a treatment plan. The careful assessment of the effect of therapy and a willingness to consider alternatives if the current plan fails are a good example of empirical scientific method. In this sense, the assessment of response to treatment becomes part of the assessment of pain.

REFERENCES

1. Bieri D, Reeve RA, Champion GD, Addicoat L, Ziegler JB, 1990 The faces pain scale for the self-assessment of the severity of pain experienced by children: development, initial validation, and preliminary investigation for ratio scale properties. Pain 41:139
2. Brown TCK and Fisk GC Anaesthesia for children. In: Pawar D (ed) Pain management, 2nd edn. Blackwell Scientific, London, ch 8, pp 127–137

11 Safety and monitoring of analgesic techniques

Philip Ragg

INTRODUCTION

The safe provision of analgesia for children requires appropriate staffing, facilities, equipment, and protocols for management. The wide range of ages, procedures, and patient conditions makes the safe provision of pain relief a challenge. Developmental changes during infancy and childhood include changes in behavior, communication (see Ch. 2), and response to drugs. An understanding of these variations will help to make the provision of analgesia appropriate. Protocols for pain management suitable for adults will usually need to be modified for children.

PRINCIPLES OF SAFE ANALGESIA FOR CHILDREN

Both the efficacy and safety of analgesia should be monitored. Monitoring protocols should specify not only the nature and frequency of observations but also reportable observations and who to inform. Staff must not only make and record observations but also understand their significance and know when to seek assistance. Medical staff must provide adequate support when problems are reported.

A number of general aspects of analgesic delivery contribute to its safe administration.

1. *Careful patient selection*: The analgesic technique chosen must be appropriate for the developmental age of the patient and for the surgery performed. More complex analgesic regimens including invasive techniques such as epidural infusions must have the consent of parents.
2. *Education*: Continuing in-service education of medical and nursing staff is essential, with provision for interaction between supervisors and practitioners. Newer analgesic regimens such as patient-controlled analgesia are also dependent upon parental and child education for their safety. Not only is education needed for the practical management of techniques but expectations of pain relief must be realistic and clear.
3. *Full documentation of techniques*: Protocols must be clear, and management must include the recording of pain, vital signs, sedation, ventilation, and complications.

4. *Appointment of personnel responsible for overseeing the management of patients*: Patients should ideally be followed up by the same team or individual to ensure continuity of care.
5. *Emergency management protocols*: Contingency plans should be clear and staff must always be available for the immediate management of complications of analgesia which can be life-threatening.
6. *Regular audit*: It is important that doctors and nurses looking after children as well as their advisers (an acute pain management team) have feedback about patient treatment so that appropriate modifications of management can be made (see Ch. 23).

STAFFING AND EDUCATION

Staff managing children with postoperative or other acute pain must be competent and adequately trained. The introduction of new analgesic techniques will require in-service training to ensure that staff have the necessary knowledge and practical skills to enable them to provide safe and effective pain management (see Ch. 12).

There should be enough trained staff to observe and assess patients regularly. Actual numbers will depend on several factors: the condition of the patients, the extent of surgery, anesthetic complications, and the quality of other assistance available. Parents may play an invaluable supportive role but are not a substitute for adequate staffing.

Staff managing children with acute pain should at all times be able to contact an appropriate medical staff member to discuss or assist with management of analgesia or complications.

LOCATION AND EQUIPMENT FOR ANALGESIC MANAGEMENT

Opinions vary regarding the appropriate location for management of children with analgesic regimens other than simple oral agents. Some anesthesiologists and intensive care specialists believe that any child being given an opioid should be managed in an intensive care unit (ICU) or high dependency unit (HDU). Others believe that this is not necessary. The two major advantages of an ICU or HDU are continuous monitoring of vital functions (respiratory and cardiac) and a high ratio of nursing staff to patients. The disadvantages are that access to these facilities may be limited and high dependency beds are more costly. Children find these units more threatening because they are noisy, less friendly, and interaction with their families is more difficult. Provided that the guidelines below are followed, it is usually safe to manage children in general wards with staff properly trained in analgesic techniques.[1]

Resuscitation equipment

Resuscitation equipment must be immediately available when a patient is using any analgesic regimen other than simple oral or nonsedative analgesics. Box 11.1 summarizes the equipment required.

Box 11.1   Equipment necessary for safe analgesic delivery

- Oxygen outlet, face masks and catheters
- Ventilation equipment (breathing systems for different ages including masks, airways, tubing, bags)
- Suction equipment and a power unit for each patient
- Intravenous equipment including cannulae, needles, syringes, infusion sets, burettes, and solutions
- Adequate lighting
- Alarm system and call for assistance button
- Monitoring equipment including pulse oximeter, blood pressure manometer (automated or manual), thermometer, stethoscopes, and electrocardiogram
- Readily available endotracheal intubation and defibrillation equipment

---

Resuscitation drugs   Drugs for the management of cardiac and respiratory depression or arrest, hypotension, arrhythmias, and local anesthetic and opioid toxicity must be immediately available in the ward. Emergency drugs recommended are listed in Box 11.2.

Box 11.2   Emergency drugs

Epinephrine (adrenaline)	Steroids
Atropine	Antihistamines
Bretylium	Succinylcholilne (suxamethonium)
Magnesium	Salbutamol
Sodium bicarbonate	Anticonvulsants
Calcium	Antiemetics
Lidocaine (lignocaine)	Naloxone
Adenosine	Flumazenil
Beta-blocker (e.g. esmolol)	

PROTOCOLS FOR MONITORING

Monitoring standards are established to safeguard against complications of analgesic delivery. Protocols are used to standardize minimum orders for a given analgesic technique. There is no substitute for vigilance by nursing and medical staff, education, familiarity with a patient's condition and the analgesic technique, and – most importantly – communication between all staff involved in the child's care. Support for ward staff must always be available for consultation about pain management problems and emergency resuscitation.

General monitoring   Minimum monitoring observations for most analgesic techniques include those listed in Box 11.3. Most of the observations should be performed hourly. Blood pressure may be recorded 4-hourly if the patient is clinically stable and at low risk of cardiovascular problems. Temperature should be measured as dictated by the patient's general condition.

Observation limits above and below which medical staff must be notified should be specified. This procedure will be facilitated by having a standard form for each analgesia technique. This form should include not

---

Box 11.3   Minimum observations for analgesic techniques

Conscious state   Temperature
Respiratory rate and depth   Patient color
Heart rate   Pain assessment
Blood pressure   Drug delivery

---

only patient details and drug prescription but also spaces that must be filled in by the prescriber specifying reportable limits for pulse rate, blood pressure, and respiratory rate, and notifiable observations specific to the technique, such as signs of local anesthetic toxicity in patients receiving local anesthetic infusions. Surgical and medical monitoring requirements such as drain tube losses or pupillary reactivity should be included when appropriate. The form should include details of other reportable observations, such as changes in conscious state or equipment malfunction and whom to contact and how to contact them. Some typical reportable observations are listed in Box 11.4.

Box 11.4   Some notifiable observations. The 'limits' (high and low) should be specified for each patient. For blood pressure, systolic, diastolic, or mean should be specified. Other notifiable observations will depend on the patient's clinical condition and the analgesia technique

Blood pressure limits $SaO_2 < 94\%$
Heart rate limits   Inadequate analgesia
Respiratory rate limits   Abnormal conscious state
Respiratory depression or difficulty   Equipment malfunction

High risk patients

Continuous pulse oximetry is recommended for high-risk patients receiving parenteral opioid analgesia. Box 11.5 lists clinical factors associated with a high risk of the respiratory complications of opioids. Box 11.6 lists indications for 'spot' pulse oximetry. Supplementary oxygen should be administered if the hemoglobin oxygen saturation falls below 94%. Medical consultation should be sought if oxygen therapy is commenced.

Box 11.5   High risk patients – continuous pulse oximetry recommended

Age less than 6 months
Concurrent use of sedative agents
Excess sedation
Sleep apnea or snoring, or airway obstruction
Spot oximetry less than 94% SaO_2
Any patient receiving supplementary oxygen
Significant cardiorespiratory impairment
Other medical indications

Opioid infusions (including PCA)

Minimum observations as outlined above and in Box 11.3 should be performed for children on opioid infusions.

A simple sedation score (e.g. 1, awake; 2, drowsy; 3, asleep) should also be recorded hourly. Complications associated with the use of opioids

---

Box 11.6   Clinical indications for 'spot' pulse oximetry

Tachypnea
Bradypnea
Respiratory distress
Breathlessness
Suspected cyanosis or impaired oxygenation
Confusion or agitation
Depressed conscious state
Hypotension

---

should be documented (e.g. nausea, vomiting, pruritus, urinary retention, constipation, agitation). The amount of opioid delivered (volume and syringe changes) must be recorded hourly, as should any change in infusion rate or boluses given.

Clear instructions regarding reportable observations and treatment of opioid toxicity including naloxone dosage and resuscitation should be recorded on the patient's chart.

Intravenous opioid bolus administration

A protocol for the administration of an intravenous opioid bolus and subsequent monitoring of the child is given in Chapter 5. The observations as described in Box 11.3 should be performed every 5 minutes for 20 minutes.

Epidural infusions

The epidural infusion chart should include details of the patient's weight and age, operation performed and epidural data (level of insertion, complications, local anesthetic drug concentration, dosage and time administered, addition of opioid and rate of infusion).

Observations

Routine: Regular observations as described above should be performed during epidural infusions of local anesthetic solution. If a dermatomal distribution of the block can be assessed, this should be routinely checked twice daily or whenever there is a clinical suspicion of excessive or inadequate neural blockade. Absence of leg weakness or presence of movement is a useful indicator that the epidural blockade is not excessive if a caudal, lumbar or low thoracic catheter is in use. Guidelines for using pulse oximetry as described above for high-risk patients (Boxes 11.5 and 11.6) may be applied to patients receiving epidural infusions. Patients receiving epidural opioids are more likely to require pulse oximetry. In some centers all children who receive epidural morphine are monitored until 12 hours after the last dose, because of its long duration of action and the risk of late respiratory depression.

As well as the observations listed in Box 11.4, signs of local anesthetic toxicity such as perioral paresthesia, tinnitus, twitching or arrhythmia, and signs of high epidural blockade such as weakness or sensory disturbance in the arms, should be listed for notification. Loss of intravenous access should be reported, as access must be maintained for the duration of the epidural infusion.

Following an epidural bolus: After an epidural bolus of local anesthetic solution, the heart rate, respiratory rate, blood pressure, and level of epidural blockade (if possible) should be assessed every 5 minutes for 20 minutes. The anesthesiologist must remain with the patient during this 20 minute period. Thereafter routine observations should be performed.

Following an increase in epidural infusion rate: After an increase in epidural infusion rate, observations as in Box 11.3 should be performed at 10 minutes, then hourly for 4 hours. The level of epidural blockade should be checked (if possible) with each of these sets of observations before reverting to routine observations.

CONCLUSION

Standard monitoring protocols and charts, careful patient selection and staff training, and appropriate consultant and resuscitation support can minimize the risks and consequences of complications of acute pain management.

REFERENCE

1. Beasley S, Tibballs J, 1987 Efficacy and safety of continuous morphine infusion for post operative analgesia in the paediatric surgical ward. Australia and NZ Journal of Surgery: 57:233–237

FURTHER READING

Gravenstein J, Paulus D 1987 Perspectives on monitoring. In: Gravenstein J, Paulus D (eds) Clinical monitoring practice. JB Lippincott, Washington ch 1, pp 1–11
US Department of Health and Human Services 1992 Acute pain management in infants, children and adolescents: operative and medical procedures. Publ. no 92–0070. Rockville

12 Nurse organization and training

Kate Brereton

INTRODUCTION

The most important nurse for a child in hospital is the one looking after that child. A nurse is the 24 hours a day presence on the ward, who is immediately responsible for the minute-to-minute assessment and care of the child and who is the link between the child and the rest of the hospital staff. The child may be in an adult referral hospital specialist ward, a district hospital (adult) general surgical ward, or a referral pediatric centre. The goals of the training of nurses should be that the nurses in each of these hospitals should be confident that they can assess a child's pain and deliver both pharmacological and nonpharmacological pain management. Each hospital should be organized so that consultation about analgesia problems is readily available. To achieve these goals requires attention to basic nurse education during training, continuing education, local hospital protocols, staffing, and clear understandings of nursing and medical responsibilities. In the different hospital environments the aims are much the same but the details of the solutions are likely to differ. Supervising staff must recognize that these aims are important and create an organization where they can be achieved.

The principles of adult education[1] apply to nurse education in pediatric pain management. The students (who may be senior staff members or college trainees) need to take responsibility for their own education, including goals and methods, while fulfilling their professional responsibilities. Ideally, within the constraints of the system, the organization and educators should try to integrate their goals and methods of training to suit those of the trainees. The clinical experience, personality, beliefs, methods, motives, and goals of both teacher and student will need to be considered to optimize learning.

QUALIFICATION-BASED NURSE TRAINING

Whether based on a hospital certificate or tertiary degree, the basic nursing qualification should include material covering pain assessment and the principles of pain management. Most of these courses will have a pediatric component, in which the differences between adult and pediatric pain management should be highlighted. Historically, course organizers structured their curriculum around established medical and nursing practice and specialities. If no department was responsible for pain management and the established departments did not consider pain management a core part of their practice, it was common for training in this area to be omitted. Similar comments apply to specialist postgraduate pediatric diplomas. Fortunately, many nursing courses now include pain management.

CONTINUING NURSE EDUCATION

Clinical nursing staff need continuing education in the area of pain management. The requirements of different staff on the same ward may be different. Deficiencies in basic training ('They didn't teach that in my day'), the introduction of new assessment or pain management techniques, transfer to a new hospital or subspeciality area, or perceived problems in daily ward management may prompt staff to pursue further training. Nursing management and educators can organize education resources and protocols for the introduction of new equipment and techniques, orientation of new staff and systems for reaccreditation to ensure that many of these education needs are met routinely.

The type of learning experience that will best fulfill the individual staff member's needs will depend on the student, the available information sources, the teacher (if one is involved), and the type of information required. Updates for those who did not receive formal basic training may be best presented in seminar or short course format, usually supplemented by personal reading. The introduction of new techniques may be best organized on a ward-by-ward basis. Care should be taken that all staff have an opportunity to attend training sessions and that written material is available on the ward as a continuing resource.

Peer support groups can provide continuing education, review, and professional support. These groups involve regular meetings of nurses, perhaps from different clinical environments, to discuss pain management problems. These may assist in communicating successful approaches to difficult problems, assure the staff that they are not alone in dealing with these issues, and can be the basis for lobbying for what may be significant changes to previous hospital nursing and medical practice. A common example would be the realization that the hospital does not have an adequate referral or consultation system for pain management problems. Solving this may involve a major change in the organization of the hospital for both nursing and medical staff.

ACCREDITATION

Core information required for accreditation for nursing supervision of specialized techniques such as epidural infusions, patient-controlled analgesia or nitrous oxide administration may best be presented in learning packages. These are a standard syllabus covering the theory, practice, and hospital protocols for each technique. The material will include information, explanation, and assessment sections. The trainees must satisfy the supervisor, usually by written or oral projects or examinations, that they have covered the work, as well as demonstrate competence at practical clinical skills. An abbreviated reaccreditation process should be a regular requirement, approximately every 2–3 years or with the introduction of new techniques or protocols.

THE ROLE OF AN ACUTE PAIN MANAGEMENT SERVICE

An acute pain management service (APMS) is pivotal in staff education, usually organizing most of the nursing education in pain management for the hospital. An experienced nurse with a combined clinical, educational, and administrative role, with suitable medical support, has a key role in an APMS. A referral pediatric center APMS can act as a resource for peripheral centers with small pediatric practices, as well as providing material for nurse training institutions, seminars, and courses. The difference in back-up in areas such as pediatric resuscitation in different hospitals must be carefully analyzed before applying protocols from referral centers to peripheral hospitals. The development of an APMS is discussed in Chapter 23.

NURSING AND MEDICAL ORGANIZATION

The situation of a child with inadequately managed pain being looked after by a nurse who identifies the problem but cannot adequately manage it can arise from a failure of organization at many levels. The nurse may not have adequate training or access to protocols on the ward, a problem that the measures described above should prevent. The numbers, training, or experience of other ward nursing staff may be insufficient to provide guidance for the less experienced staff member. The medical staff responsible for the patient may not be consulted or may not respond to the problem adequately. The medical staff may have analogous training and referral problems. Clearly, both medical and nursing staff need to be equally well organized, trained and committed. In the absence of an APMS, a particular group such as an anesthesia department can be assigned responsibility for receiving referrals concerning pain management problems from the medical staff directly associated with the patient. The patient's medical staff may then perceive consultation as a routine interdepartmental referral rather than an admission of failure.

Modern business management has highlighted the concept that an organization can have a 'culture'. The nursing and medical education and organization described above may constitute a major change in some hospitals. In these hospitals, successful implementation of modern pain management may require a new culture rather than new equipment.

REFERENCE

1. Brundage DH, MacKeracher D 1980. Adult learning principles and their application to program planning. Ontario Ministry of Education, Institute for Studies in Education, Toronto

13 Nonpharmacological pain management

Kate Brereton

INTRODUCTION

Nonpharmacological pain management techniques may be general – how the child and family are 'handled' physically and emotionally – or specific, or both. Commonly, these techniques are used to supplement rather than replace pharmacological management of acute pain in hospital. Conversely, pharmacological treatment will usually be more effective when combined with these techniques.

It is widely agreed that 'simple' comforting can provide relief to an injured child. The mechanisms by which comforting may relieve pain are worth bearing in mind when any analgesic technique is applied. Many 'simple' steps may contribute to the process. The child may be relieved that help is at hand, physically comforted by cradling and immobilization of an injured part, reassured that their problem is addressed ('Where does it hurt?') and a plan is in place ('I'll take you home and bandage it'), and assisted by counterstimuli (stroking the head, holding the child's hand, talking or singing) and distraction (drawing attention to something in the immediate environment). The details of what will be effective for a particular child will vary with developmental stage, personality, family, staff, the injury, and the environment. This is the art of patient care. The psychology and physiology of 'simple' comforting can be analyzed in much greater depth and detail, but the message is clear: a hospital environment that does not have a 'culture' of caring for children will be less likely to succeed in delivering analgesia.

An illustration may help demonstrate the importance of the 'art' of patient care. Perhaps the correct management of a patient's pain involves increasing the rate of a morphine infusion already in place and giving a bolus of the morphine. This simple change could be a prompt response to a patient's changing analgesic requirements, accompanied by a quick check that the pain is not a sign of a new condition. A few words of explanation, review of other patient needs, reassurance that the patient will be reviewed later but can call again if necessary, and a suggestion of a suitable activity (reading to the child, drawing, television as appropriate) complete a brief but effective response. This scenario will most probably produce a satisfied, undistressed patient, even if the morphine needs to be increased later. In contrast, the same pharmacological change made by someone who is rushed and seems insensitive to the patient and family needs may exacerbate any anxieties, anger, and sense of helplessness felt by the patient (and family). This may be sufficient to turn a potentially effective morphine dose into an ineffective one, and may discourage future requests for pain relief. There are substantial benefits from an organized professional approach to pain management.

Although complete relief of acute pain may often be achieved, acceptance that reasonable control of pain is the aim of treatment can be an important step in pain management. An unrealistic expectation of perfect pain control will usually lead to disappointment. The natural history of most acute pain is for it to resolve. The patient or family may feel reassured that the plan is to keep the patient comfortable until he or she gets better, rather than to expect a pain-free course, or become anxious that the presence of any pain represents a serious pathological condition that must be eliminated. Similarly, any new analgesic therapy should be introduced as something that may lessen rather than eliminate pain.

Staff should be sensitive to the wishes and circumstances of each patient and family, recognizing that they may have specific anxieties or concerns about some of these therapies. No therapy should be undertaken without willing, informed agreement by the patient and family. Formal written consent may be unnecessary for many of the therapies described, although nursing staff should ensure that their practice is within their hospital's nursing code of conduct.

Prompt, effective pain management can prevent a 'vicious circle' of fear and anxiety exacerbating pain, and prevent long-term maladaptive behavioral responses,[1,2] such as introversion, nightmares, and enuresis. There are many specific nonpharmacological techniques, some of which are briefly discussed below, but the key to successful pain control is a personal relationship with the child (and family) and repeated pain assessments which prompt appropriate action in a caring environment. A number of techniques may be suitable for a particular child. Staff should use a suitable technique with which they are comfortable and refer when appropriate.

PSYCHOLOGICAL TECHNIQUES

Psychological techniques must be appropriate to the developmental stage, personality, and circumstances of the patient. Education and explanation of the nature of the child's pain management and pathology may assist some patients to cope (others may prefer 'not to know'), while control of anxiety is an important supplement to pain control for most patients.

The parents of infants may need help in controlling their own anxiety, to prevent this being transmitted to and unsettling their children. Parents can learn techniques that staff use to assist their children and should be asked by staff what methods have previously been used by that family. Older children often respond well to techniques that increase their sense of self-control, such as training in relaxation techniques, breathing control, and autohypnosis. An episode of loss of control can cause long-term erosion of the self-esteem of an adolescent. These methods may be particularly useful for the control of minor procedural pain. Preparation for the procedure may involve formal training in a psychological pain control technique.

Some formal psychological techniques will require specially trained staff and are particularly suited to recurrent acute procedural pain or chronic pain. In these circumstances, it is more likely that the time and effort required to teach the technique will be adequately rewarded. If a patient is to be trained in a formal psychological technique, it may be necessary to find a suitable area where the training can be done away from the distractions of the hospital ward. The area should be comfortable and quiet with adequate space for the patient, teacher, appropriate family members, and staff involved in the patient's care.

Distraction

Distraction is perhaps the simplest and most widely used psychological technique. The child's pain experience is minimized by focusing attention elsewhere. Any of the senses and any combination of senses may be involved, while the child's attention may be held by a story, activities, or imagined sensations. This overlaps with other techniques (see below) such as play, music, and imaging. It is particularly useful for minimizing the distress of painful procedures. Timing of the distraction in relation to the procedure is important, as the child's pain may return if the distraction finishes before the procedure.

Breathing techniques

Training in controlled breathing can induce relaxation, provide a focus for distraction, be part of an imaging technique or be used as a simple form of biofeedback. The breathing pattern will usually be rhythmic and must be sustainable. Breathing at approximately normal tidal volume and rate is usually the most comfortable.

Progressive muscle relaxation

To achieve relaxation, the child can be taught progressive deliberate relaxation of the body part by part. Some variants involve tensing the part before letting it go limp, 'like a rag doll'. Initially a staff member instructs the child as each part of the procedure is performed. A parent may take over the role of instructor and many children will rapidly learn to use the technique independently.

Meditation

Meditation is a useful strategy for treating anxiety and improving the child's internal coping mechanisms. One technique uses focused awareness of breathing. The presence of acute pain may make it more difficult to achieve a meditative state, the lack of other distractions potentially creating a focus of attention on the pain.

Imagery

Imagery includes a number of more formal distraction techniques. The child may imagine something pleasant, be drawn by a 'guide' through an imagined scene, or specifically be asked to visualize things that will lessen their pain. The process should involve multiple senses. Imagery can be difficult to use in children under 3 years old as their attention span is limited. Adolescents are more likely to require structured externally guided images to enter an appropriate mental state.[3,4]

Hypnotherapy

Although emphasis is often placed on the power of suggestion during hypnotic states, this state of mind has much in common with those produced by other formal relaxation and imaging techniques. Some would describe these techniques as a form of hypnosis. Autohypnosis has been used in the control of chronic and procedural pain. Hypnosis is being used with increasing frequency in children.

Biofeedback

Biofeedback involves giving the subjects immediate information about a physiological parameter, such as heart rate, blood pressure, respiratory rate, or electromyographic measures of muscle tension, allowing the subjects to train themselves to consciously control what are normally involuntary bodily functions. The values fed back usually relate to a bodily function that will change with anxiety-related autonomic activity. The feedback both alerts the subject that stress is occurring and improves stress control by the now conscious control of the physiological changes associated with stress. This control of stress improves pain relief.

Music therapy

Music can be a useful tool for distraction, entertainment, relaxation, and expression for children. The child can be active (making or choosing music) or passive (listening to music). Many pediatric centers now have trained paramedical music therapists, but nursing and paramedical staff frequently use these techniques.

Play therapy

Like music, play can provide distraction, entertainment, relaxation, and expression, but is especially useful for the educational preparation of young children for procedures. These children are likely to express their fears and fantasies about the procedure via play, especially using dolls to model their patient role[3,5] (see also Ch. 20, 'Intravenous cannulation'). Again, many pediatric centers now have trained paramedical play therapists.

Aromatherapy

Aromatherapy uses the scents of essential oils extracted from plants. These methods may improve the ambience of the hospital environment, provide some positive sensory distraction from pain,[6] and can be combined with physical therapies such as massage. Used correctly, complications of this therapy are very rare.

Tactile therapy

Tactile therapy includes a wide range of treatments using touch. The role, mechanisms, and methods vary in this complex group of treatments.

Simple human comforting by touch has obvious efficacy in assisting pain control. Physiological effects are well documented and can depend on the psychological state of both patient and 'therapist' and on their relationship. There is also a wide spectrum of tactile therapy involved with therapeutic touch,[7] massage, manipulation and mobilization, and acupressure. Cutaneous stimulation may cause inhibition of pain impulse transmission at a spinal level and perception at a cortical level. These techniques are often helpful even if the mechanisms of action are uncertain.

Debriefing

Debriefing involves a formal discussion of the pros and cons and reasons behind a particular clinical sequence of events, not only to learn from those events but also to allow venting of emotions and plans for the future to be made. Staff, the patient, and the family may be involved, although sessions with staff alone may be useful. Debriefing is of particular importance for a patient if a distressing pain experience occurs, especially if the pain was due to a procedure which will need to be repeated. Staff may benefit from debriefing, both to help them come to terms with distress due to the clinical course of a patient, and to highlight successful techniques.

Affirmations

Patients can be guided to replace the negative meanings they have given their pain with more positive self-statements and meanings.[3,8] Such affirmations can be recorded on an audiotape with accompanying relaxation music.

Role models

The child can be encouraged to observe or interact with a peer who has encountered a similar situation and mastered effective and appropriate coping skills. The role model involved should not endeavor to show the other child that there is no pain or distress associated with the procedure, but rather that strategies can be used to manage it. By using peer support and guidance the child can gain confidence to develop an individual coping style.[3]

Journalling

Patients keep a diary noting pain intensity and nature, the feelings it evokes, precipitating factors, what they did to cope with it, and their pain management goals. This offers children a structured outlet to explore their inner feelings and the meanings and associations they have attached to their pain experience. It is also a way for them to evaluate their plan of action and their self-management skills.[9] This technique is mainly of use in chronic pain management in older children.

PHYSICAL METHODS

As described above for tactile therapy, hands-on physical therapy covers a wide range of treatments, while thermal, electrical, and other forms of energy can also be used. Most pediatric centers will have physiotherapists both to manage patients and to advise and train other staff, patients, and parents, about appropriate physical therapies.

Acute soft tissue injuries, including sports injuries and some surgical procedures, are initially treated with: rest, ice, compression, and elevation, (RICE). These methods tend to reduce pain by minimizing edema which stretches tissues and contains inflammatory mediators. The trend these days is for early mobilization to prevent disuse changes and to speed rehabilitation. This may need to be supported by increased pharmacological analgesia, if initiated within days of the injury or surgery. There are often psychological and practical benefits in training the child (and/or family) in the application of physical methods.[5]

Immobilization

Immobilization is particularly indicated for acute conditions where further injury (and pain) will result from movement of the injured part. An excellent example is the relief of the pain of fractures by splinting. Immobilization with plasters, traction or slings rather than with internal fixation or external fixateurs is the preferred treatment of many fractures in childhood. This is because of the moulding and rapid healing of bone in young children combined with their resistance to prolonged problems with disuse atrophy.

Cryotherapy

Ice packs for acute injury cause vasoconstriction, lessen edema, slow chemical reactions (such as inflammatory reactions), and reduce nerve conduction velocity and activity which may reduce pain. Freezing destroys tissue, and should be avoided by limiting the duration of exposure and by not using very low temperature applications. Some children, especially younger ones, will not tolerate the discomfort of an extremely cold stimulus, making cryotherapy unsuitable.[5]

Heat therapy

Mild heat therapy can relieve muscle spasm and joint stiffness, especially in chronic inflammatory states. Heat may help the mobilization phase of rehabilitation after acute injury. Thermal injury should be avoided by supervision and careful selection of the heat source, the temperature and the duration of therapy. Sensory deficit (e.g. following local anesthetic block) is a relative contraindication to heat therapy as the warning pain of tissue damage will be absent.

Massage

Massage may have many roles (see above). Massage of the acutely injured or inflamed part is relatively contraindicated. Classically, massage is used as part of the mobilization process, after the acute phase. Muscle spasm can be decreased and edema fluid mobilized. Organizing hematoma and adhesions may also be broken down. There are also potential benefits in the human touch and therapeutic relationship (as above), and spinal inhibition of pain transmission from cutaneous and proprioceptive stimulation away from the painful area.[10] Older children can learn to perform their own massage. Many of these general benefits should occur whatever type of massage therapy (e.g. relaxation, remedial, aromatherapy, or shiatsu) is being used.

Therapeutic exercises

Therapeutic exercises may be specifically designed to speed mobilization and rehabilitation of an acutely injured area. Exercises may also be used to prevent and reverse the impact of disuse on the uninjured part of the body. Children who are expected to have a difficult or prolonged rehabilitation phase may benefit from a personal structured program supervised by a physiotherapist. The aim is increasing activity without increasing pain, while the shortening of the rehabilitation period should decrease pain.

Ultrasound

Ultrasound can be used during rehabilitation after acute injury to produce deep tissue heating and increase blood flow. Its use is contraindicated in children whose growth plates are not closed.[11]

Transcutaneous electrical nerve stimulation

Transcutaneous electrical nerve stimulation (TENS) has mainly been used in the rehabilitation phase of acute injury and for chronic pain. Adhesive skin electrodes are placed usually over the painful site, and the current flow is increased until a tolerable tingling sensation is produced. Various regimens for the duration of each therapy are used. Many patients are trained to use this technique at home. Analgesia may result from spinal nerve stimulation, producing spinal inhibition of pain impulse transmission or endorphin release.[12,13]

Acupuncture

Originating from traditional Chinese medicine, with its theory of meridians and points on the body having influence over specific organs and mental states, acupuncture is widely used in Western medicine. The insertion of needles, with or without low or high frequency electrical stimulation, is not a process that children readily accept. Acupressure, using local pressure rather than needles at the appropriate points, may be an alternative or supplement, but is less effective. The advent of laser acupuncture has made the technique much more acceptable to children. A narrow beam (about 3 mm) laser is used virtually painlessly to stimulate the selected point. The laser may induce a peculiar sensation at the site of application which is usually not interpreted as pain. There is evidence that acupuncture works by the release of endogenous opioid peptides.[14]

EVALUATION

The efficacy of nonpharmacological techniques should receive the same scrutiny as pharmacological techniques. The patient should have developmentally appropriate pain assessment before and after the treatment or course of treatment. Decreased anxiety or improved sleep patterns or behavior may be sufficient indication for continuation of some of these therapies, even if there is little change in the formal pain assessment. Continuing therapy also requires cooperation of the child and family, without which even an apparently effective therapy may need to be withdrawn.

CONCLUSION

Nonpharmacological treatment has a major role in the management of pain. Simple common-sense psychological and physical comforting of children in pain should be part of routine treatment. More sophisticated techniques can extend the role of nonpharmacological analgesia if the resources and trained personnel are available.

REFERENCES

1. Baker C, Wong D 1987 QUEST A process of pain assessment in children. Orthopaedic Nursing 6:11–19.
2. Broome M 1990 Preparation of children for painful procedures. Paediatric Nursing 16:537–541
3. Patterson K, Ware L 1988 Coping skills for children undergoing painful medical procedures. Issues in Comprehensive Paediatric Nursing 11:113–143
4. McCaffery M, Beebe A 1989 Pain, a clinical manual for nursing practice. CV Mosby, St Louis, pp 212, 294
5. Eland J 1990 Pain in children. Symptom management. Nursing Clinics of North America 25:871–882
6. Tisserand R 1989 The art of aromatherapy. CW Daniel, Saffron Walden, UK, pp 13–16.
7. Jurgens A, Meehan TC, Wilson HL 1987 Therapeutic touch as a nursing intervention. Holistic Nursing Practice, 2:1–13
8. Hay L 1988 You can heal your life. Specialist Publications, Concord, NSW, pp 82, 95–96.
9. Keefe FJ, Lefabure JC 1994 Behaviour Therapy. In: Melzack R, Wall PD (eds) Textbook of Pain, 3rd edn. Churchill Livingstone, Edinburgh, pp 1371–1373
10. Carter B 1994 Child and infant pain. Principles of nursing care and management. Chapman & Hall, London pp 95–96
11. Houck C, Troshynski T, Berde C 1994 Treatment of pain in children. In: Melzack R, Wall PD, (eds) Textbook of Pain, 3rd edn. Churchill Livingstone, Edinburgh p 1428
12. North R 1994 Handbook of Pain Management, 2nd edn. Williams & Wilkins, Baltimore, p 75
13. Woolf CJ, Thompson JW 1994 Stimulation-induced analgesia: transcutaneous electrical nerve stimulation (TENS) and vibration. In: Textbook of pain, 3rd edn. Churchill Livingstone, Edinburgh, pp 1191–1192
14. Editorial, British Medical Journal 1981, 283:746–747

14 Management of common problems

Philip Ragg, Ian McKenzie

INTRODUCTION

Successful pain management in children can usually be achieved with few complications. The choice of analgesia is made by weighing up the advantages and disadvantages of the available methods for that patient. A number of children will present with problems relating to their pain management. The origin (diagnosis) of the problem should be carefully assessed by the usual clinical methods, particularly history and examination. Accurate diagnosis should lead to appropriate medical or surgical treatment. If the problem appears to be due to the analgesic technique, consideration should be given to modifying the technique, trying a different technique, or symptomatic treatment.

This chapter outlines the management of some common problems that may involve or complicate pain management. The problems discussed are inadequate analgesia, nausea and vomiting, respiratory depression, pruritus, urinary retention, agitation, and constipation.

INADEQUATE ANALGESIA

There are a number of steps in assessing and managing a patient who appears to have inadequate analgesia. A careful history is the most important step in pain management. A number of questions must be answered.

- What is the cause of the pain? The nature, site, and associated features of the pain will usually limit the number of likely diagnoses. For postoperative patients it is important not to assume that the pain is due to 'usual' postoperative pain and simply increase the analgesia dose. Pain from other sources or complications of surgery may need specific therapeutic intervention. Tight plasters require elevation of the limb and possibly splitting of the plaster. Urinary retention may need passage of a urethral catheter. Intermittent pain due to muscle spasm may require antispasmodics.

A problem that is common in pediatrics is the distressed, crying infant or young child who has a potential source of pain (such as following an operation), who also has many possible sources of distress other than pain, such as hunger, exhaustion, anger, disruption of routine, or parental separation. Treatment will often need to be a 'best guess', having considered the possibilities. It is important to review the success of this management. Sensitive explanation of the reasons for the management plan and the promise of follow-up will often help reassure the family that the child's distress is being taken seriously. Occasionally, especially in the evening after an operation, staff may recognize when young children are simply very angry at not being at home and taking part in their usual routine. The suggestion of this diagnosis is sometimes greeted with relief by the family who may recognize the behavior but assume that it is due to pain.

- What analgesia has already been given and why is it inadequate? If analgesia is inadequate it is commonly because either an inappropriate regimen was chosen (see Ch. 15 for suggested regimens for common operations) or that the regimen chosen has not been applied properly. Another reason is that a new pain stimulus that needs specific treatment may have arisen, such as pressure within a plaster cast or wound infection.

Answering the following questions may help to solve common problems in pain management.

- Is the diagnosis of the cause of the pain correct and the treatment appropriate?
- Has the correct dose of acetaminophen (paracetamol) been given and continued? (Remember the rectal route.)
- Has a local anesthetic block regressed, requiring initiation of alternative pain management?
- Have oral or rectal opioids or NSAIDs been used and, if so, was the dose appropriate? These drugs may be especially useful in a patient without intravenous access.
- Has an opioid infusion been appropriately titrated to the patient's needs and have boluses been used to attain therapeutic blood levels? (Changing the infusion rate alone produces slow changes in blood levels, see Ch. 5.)
- If using patient-controlled analgesia (PCA), does the patient understand the system and have confidence to use it correctly? Check the actual amount of drug administered.
- If PCA is used, are the bolus and lockout times appropriate? Is a background infusion required, and if so, what dose should be prescribed? (See Ch. 6.)
- For infusion systems, is there a problem with dosage or delivery of the drug?
- For epidural and other local anesthetic infusions, is the block adequate? Would the patient benefit from a bolus of local anesthetic drug, an increased infusion rate, a change in concentration of local anesthetic solution, or a change in the position of either the patient or the catheter? (See Ch. 7.)
- Should a local anesthetic infusion which is not providing adequate analgesia be stopped, or supplemented with systemic analgesics such as acetaminophen or opioids? Often the local anesthetic infusion should be continued and low doses of other agents will be an adequate supplement.

- Would the removal of fentanyl from an epidural infusion allow safe supplementation of the block with an intravenous opioid infusion or PCA?
- Are the patient's and family's expectations of analgesia reasonable? Sometimes the presence of minimal discomfort will be poorly tolerated. Advice about the aims of the analgesia, the risks and benefits of alternative analgesia, the likely progress of the patient, general support and review will result in acceptance of less than perfect analgesia. This may be preferable to changing pharmacological treatment.
- If anxiety is exacerbating the pain response and advice and reassurance fail, is there a place for specific psychological techniques (see Ch. 13), sedation or anxiolytic medication?

NAUSEA AND VOMITING

Nausea and vomiting are often multifactorial in origin. Causes may be peripheral, central, or both, and may involve direct effects on the vomiting system together with afferent input from many other areas. Possible contributory factors are listed in Box 14.1.

Box 14.1   Factors which may contribute to nausea and vomiting:

Surgery (especially intraabdominal, orbital, ear, nose and throat, dental)
Patient sensitivity (e.g. past history of motion sickness or vomiting)
Opioid usage
Other drugs (e.g. digoxin, chemotherapeutic agents)
Gastric stasis, atony or ileus
Anxiety
Pain
Biochemical (hypoxia, hypercapnia, hypoglycemia, hyperkalemia, hypocalcemia)
Other pathology (e.g. hypotension or raised intracranial pressure)

Management

General measures

1. Cease oral intake.
2. Minimize movement of the child.
3. Encourage rest and sleep.
4. Consider intravenous fluids (for rehydration and to supply glucose to prevent or reverse ketosis).
5. Consider investigations (e.g. arterial blood gas and electrolytes) to assess the severity of the physiological disturbance caused by vomiting.

Specific measures

- Treat specific causes:
  - stop the opioid, if alternative analgesia is satisfactory
  - treat anxiety with a benzodiazepine
  - insert a nasogastric tube for bowel obstruction
- Symptomatic treatment:
  - Administer antiemetic drug intravenously or intramuscularly (see Table 14.1).

It may be appropriate to give an antiemetic for symptom control even if other specific measures are being used

All the drugs in Table 14.1 (except ondansetron and tropisetron) may rarely cause dystonic reactions, such as oculogyric crisis. This is more likely with high and repeated doses but appears to be idiosyncratic in some patients. Benztropine (0.02 mg/kg i.v. or i.m., may be repeated in 15 minutes if required) should be available for the treatment of such reactions. Blood pressure should be monitored when droperidol is given as it may cause vasodilation and hypotension due to alpha-adrenergic blockade.

Table 14.1   Antiemetic drugs and dosage

Drug	Dosage
Metoclopramide	0.15–0.25mg/kg
Droperidol	20–50 µg/kg
Prochlorperazine	0.25 mg/kg
Promethazine	0.2–0.5 mg/kg
Cyclizine	1 mg/kg
Ondansetron	100 µg/kg
Tropisetron	0.2 mg/kg

RESPIRATORY DEPRESSION

See Chapter 5 for a discussion of the use of opioids in children.

Management

- Consider diagnosis of cause of respiratory depression
- *Mild respiratory depression* (moderate decrease in respiratory rate, HbO_2 saturation decreased but greater than 90%):

  - consider decreasing or withdrawing opioid if associated with marked sedation
  - administer oxygen
  - stimulate patient
  - continuously monitor pulse oximetry, heart rate, and respiratory rate

- *Severe respiratory depression* (apnea, HbO_2 saturation less than 90% or significant decrease in respiratory rate or heart rate):

  - support airway, breathing, and circulation (ABC) as required
  - withdraw opioid
  - administer oxygen
  - naloxone 2 µg/kg increased to 100 µg/kg by doubling the dosage as required
  - summon resuscitation team
  - continuously monitor pulse oximetry, heart rate, respiratory rate and blood pressure

PRURITUS

Pruritus may be due to many different causes and consideration should be given to whether the itching is due to a local irritant or a systemic reaction such as histamine release. Some of the more common causes of pruritus are shown in Box 14.2.

Box 14.2   Pruritus: differential diagnoses

Opioids (especially morphine and epidural opioids)
Other drugs (especially those releasing histamine)
Heat or warm ambient temperature
Topical creams or lotions
Physiological causes (rash, fever, viremia)
Dermatological diseases or associations (uremia, bilirubinemia, diabetes)
Insect bites
Allergy, including anaphylaxis

Management

1. Distraction or reassurance may be helpful
2. The itching may be relieved by cool sponges and topical treatment (calamine or local anesthetic solutions)
3. Change opioid (intravenous or epidural). *Note:* Pruritus is less common with fentanyl than morphine.
4. Give promethazine 200 µg/kg intravenously.
5. Epidural opioid-induced pruritus can be reversed with naloxone 5 µg/kg intravenously – this may reverse analgesia also.
6. Resuscitate as necessary for anaphylaxis.

URINARY RETENTION

Management

- *Acute or nonsevere retention:*
  - cease opioid or epidural if appropriate
  - conservative management (e.g. observation, reassurance, manual expression)
  - encouragement strategies such as privacy or running water
  - intermittent catheterization

- *Obstruction or severe retention:*
  - indwelling urinary catheter
  - consider seeking surgical or neurological consultation

AGITATION/TWITCHING

Possible causes of agitation or twitching are given in Box 14.3.

Box 14.3   Agitation: differential diagnoses

Drug reaction
Sleep deprivation
Pain
Acute brain syndrome (all causes)
Opioid toxicity (in particular normeperidine toxicity)
Local anesthetic drug toxicity

Management

1. Withdraw the opioid or drug implicated.
2. Give the reversal drug:
    a. Physostigmine for scopolamine toxicity
    b. Naloxone for opioid toxicity
    c. Flumazenil for benzodiazepine toxicity
    d. Benztropine for extrapyramidal reactions
3. Administer sedation (benzodiazepines, e.g. diazepam 0.05–0.1 mg/kg).
4. Investigate possible causes with the following tests:
    a. Electrolytes including potassium, calcium, magnesium
    b. Arterial blood gases
    c. Urea and creatinine, and liver function tests
    d. Measurement of plasma level of opioid
    e. Full blood examination

CONSTIPATION

Causes of constipation are listed in Box 14.4

Box 14.4 Constipation: differential diagnoses

Opioid side-effect
Long-term problem (past history)
Post-operative ileus
Endocrine or metabolic causes (hypokalemia, hypercalcemia)
Neurological causes (primary or secondary to epidural or caudal analgesia)
Drug causes:
  – tricyclic antidepressants
  – aluminum-containing antacids
  – iron
  – calcium antagonists
  – phenothiazines

Management

1. Withdraw opioid if appropriate
2. Surgical consultation is necessary if constipation is associated with pain, distension, or anal fissures
3. Reassure the patient
4. Increase fluids and fiber if appropriate.
5. Pharmacological treatment:
    a. Osmotic laxatives (lactulose)
    b. Stool softeners (paraffin oil)
    c. Suppositories and enemas

FURTHER READING

Gravenstein J, Paulus D 1987 Clinical monitoring practice. JB Lippincott, Washington, pp 1–11
US Department of Health and Human Services 1992. Acute pain management in infants, children and adolescents: operative and medical procedures. Publ. No. 92-0070. Rockville,
Watcha M, White P 1992 Post operative nausea and vomiting. Anaesthesiology 77:162–184.

15 Practical aspects of postoperative analgesia

Phil Gaukroger

INTRODUCTION

This chapter describes some general principles of postoperative pain management and gives appropriate regimens for analgesia for common pediatric surgical procedures. A range of suitable analgesic techniques are mentioned for most procedures, the choice depending on local preferences, training, facilities, and often the exact surgical technique used. For example, some surgeons almost never use a suprapubic urinary catheter for hypospadias repair; others will use a suprapubic catheter routinely. Analgesic requirements are usually greater in the children with suprapubic catheters. Details of the various postoperative analgesia techniques are discussed in the appropriate chapters. Further aspects of the general management of postoperative pain can be found in Chapters 11 and 14 concerning monitoring, safety, and complications of pain management.

PRINCIPLES OF POSTOPERATIVE ANALGESIA

The child and parents should be told before the operation how postoperative pain will be controlled. They need to know how long the analgesic technique is likely to be needed and what will be available when it is stopped. The explanation should leave them with realistic expectations of the efficacy of analgesia. This does much to alleviate anxiety and fear and improves the postoperative course. The psychological needs of children should be considered. Parental presence and comfort will help most children experiencing pain both in the recovery room and in the ward.

All staff caring for the patient, including anesthesiologists, surgeons, ward nursing staff, and ward medical staff should be aware of which analgesic technique is being used. With all methods, and particularly with specialized techniques, staff should be appropriately trained to avoid accidents or poor management. Pain management should not be considered in isolation, but needs to be integrated with other aspects of the child's rehabilitation after surgery such as oral intake, mobilization, and physiotherapy. Side-effects such as nausea, vomiting, pruritus, sedation, motor blockade, and urinary retention can be more troublesome than pain, and should be managed appropriately and not ignored (see Ch. 14). The surgical team should be consulted if surgical problems are suspected.

The primary responsibility for managing a child's postoperative pain may lie with the surgeon or the anesthesiologist. Postoperative pain control should be coordinated by an individual or group of individuals within the hospital. Often these include anesthetic personnel who may provide a formal acute pain management service (see also Ch. 23). This team should be involved with all patients having specialized pain treatment such as epidural infusions or patient-controlled analgesia (PCA), and should be available for consultation about other patients with problems with postoperative pain control.

Anesthesiologists should aim to have their patients awaken having already received effective analgesia, as it is more difficult to treat a child who has established pain. If intravenous opioids are going to be used intraoperatively and postoperatively, a single opioid should be used and initiated intraoperatively. If opioids are required in the recovery room they should be titrated intravenously for rapid onset.

METHODS OF ANALGESIC ADMINISTRATION IN CHILDREN

In the past, methods of drug administration were not tailored to the requirements of children. For many clinicians the only treatments for acute pain were intramuscular meperidine (pethidine) or acetaminophen (paracetamol) often in inadequate doses. Numerous surveys have demonstrated the inadequacy of pain management in the past. Children dislike intramuscular injections and this route should usually be avoided. Children may deny having pain rather than have an injection. It is essential that nonpainful methods of administration are used. The intravenous and oral routes of analgesic administration are more acceptable for most children.

Most children find oral administration acceptable unless the flavour of syrups or tablets is unpleasant. Taste is an underestimated factor in deciding which drug to prescribe. For example, morphine syrup is extremely bitter and many children reject it within a day of starting it. Acetaminophen is well accepted by most children and comes in a variety of pleasantly flavored oral preparations. Taste does not matter when drugs are given via a feeding gastrostomy or nasogastric tube. Rectal administration of loading doses of acetaminophen following induction of anesthesia causes little disturbance to the patient, minimizes the risk of expulsion, and allows adequate time for absorption.

Intermittent intravenous opioid boluses (see Ch. 5 for protocol) are the simple alternative to intermittent intramuscular injections of opioids. This technique of opioid administration is potentially labour-intensive and is best reserved for situations where pain is expected to be moderate or of short duration, for example following fractures or minor surgery. Drug calculation errors are a potential hazard when small doses of opioids are prescribed and administered in children. Patient-controlled analgesia or an intravenous opioid infusion are better methods for opioid delivery if the pain is likely to be more severe or longer-lasting; PCA is preferred in children who can manage this technique (see Ch. 6).

Local anesthetic techniques are commonly used, particularly in day surgery cases where infiltration and neural blockade allow a quick and pain-free recovery without opioid side-effects. Epidural infusions can be very effective in major abdominal and thoracic cases.

TECHNIQUES FOR MANAGING POSTOPERATIVE PAIN

There are many methods available for postoperative pain control. The aim of this section is to suggest a range of suitable analgesic techniques for specific surgical procedures, recognizing that practices vary widely.

Where practical, local anesthetic drugs should be given intraoperatively to supplement postoperative analgesia. Unless contraindicated, acetaminophen should usually be given whenever complete analgesia cannot be achieved by local anesthetic means.

Note that 'acetaminophen loading' refers to either the administration of oral acetaminophen 20 mg/kg before surgery or the administration of rectal acetaminophen 30 mg/kg following induction of anesthesia.

Analgesia for common pediatric surgical procedures

- *Circumcision:*
  - single-injection caudal block with or without acetaminophen loading; acetaminophen as needed postoperatively *or*
  - penile block with or without acetaminophen loading; acetaminophen as needed postoperatively *or*
  - application of lidocaine jelly to the wound and acetaminophen loading

- *Hypospadias:*
  - Single-injection caudal block with or without acetaminophen loading; intravenous opioids or oral acetaminophen as needed postoperatively *or*
  - continuous caudal epidural blockade for 1–3 days (for more extensive cases) *or*
  - caudal clonidine or opioid (fentanyl)

- *Ureteric reimplantation, pyeloplasty:*
  - intravenous opioid, acetaminophen loading and 'single shot' local anesthetic technique intraoperatively; postoperative PCA (no or low-dose background infusion) or i.v. opioid infusion
  - continuous epidural infusion using a bupivacaine and fentanyl mixture

- *Inguinal hernia, hydrocele, orchidopexy:*
  - acetaminophen loading plus bupivacaine 0.25% wound infiltration and ilioinguinal nerve block. Acetaminophen as needed postoperatively
  - caudal bupivacaine 0.25% 1 ml/kg plus acetaminophen loading. Acetaminophen as needed postoperatively

- *Umbilical hernia:*
  - bupivacaine 0.25% wound infiltration plus acetaminophen loading; acetaminophen as needed postoperatively

- *Open appendicectomy:*
  - acetaminophen with or without i.v. opioid loading intraoperatively (possibly wound infiltration with local anesthetic drug). Postoperative PCA (no background infusion) or i.v. opioid boluses as required, or opioid infusion then acetaminophen, *or*
  - intraoperative 11th right intercostal block plus acetaminophen loading; postoperatively, acetaminophen and i.v. opioid boluses, both as needed, or opioid infusion

- *Laparoscopic appendicectomy:*
  - intravenous opioid loading plus acetaminophen loading; postoperatively, opioid boluses and acetaminophen, both as needed

- *Laparotomy:*
  - intraoperative acetaminophen and i.v. opioid loading; postoperative PCA with background infusion or, if unsuitable for PCA, opioid infusion; oral analgesics when taking oral fluids, *or*
  - epidural infusion with 0.125% bupivacaine alone or with fentanyl

- *Neonatal laparotomy or ligation of patent ductus arteriosus:*
  - intraoperative fentanyl loading (2–5 μg/kg if planning to extubate;10–50 μg/kg if child to be ventilated); and acetaminophen loading; postoperative low-dose morphine infusion (up to 20 μg/kg per hour). Nurse and monitor in appropriate area. Intercostal blocks or wound infiltration with local anesthetic agent may be used

- *Pyloromyotomy:*
  - wound infiltration and acetaminophen loading; acetaminophen as needed postoperatively

- *Lacerations, foreign bodies, abscess, lymph node biopsy, etc:*
  - intraoperative acetaminophen loading alone or with bupivacaine 0.25% wound infiltration; acetaminophen as needed postoperatively

- *Thoracotomy:*
  - fentanyl or morphine loading with or without intercostal blocks intraoperatively; postoperative PCA (with background infusion) or opioid infusion, *or*
  - epidural infusion

- *Posterior spinal fusion:*
  - fentanyl or morphine loading intraoperatively; postoperative PCA (with background infusion) for 2–3 days followed by oral analgesics alone or with benzodiazepines

Note: these patients often require higher opioid doses

- *Anterior spinal fusion:*
  - fentanyl or morphine loading intraoperatively; postoperative PCA (with background infusion) for 2–3 days, then oral analgesics, *or*
  - postoperative epidural infusion

- *Fractures:*
  - preoperative and/or intraoperative opioid until comfortable; acetaminophen loading. Oral analgesia postoperatively. *Note:* femoral nerve blockade (single injection or catheter) is useful for fractured femur.

- *Lower limb surgery:*
  - postoperative PCA (no background infusion) or i.v. opioid boluses or infusion, change to oral analgesics after 1–2 days, *and/or*
  - Femoral or sciatic nerve block. If patient's leg requires plaster, discuss the risk of compartment syndrome and pressure necrosis with the surgeon. *Note:* caudal analgesia may be useful for selected cases

- *Ventilating ear tubes, antral washout, adenoidectomy, etc:*
  - acetaminophen alone or with codeine loading preoperatively; acetaminophen as required after procedure

- *Tonsillectomy:*
  - acetaminophen loading and 0.05–0.15 mg/kg morphine intraoperatively; acetaminophen 4-hourly postoperatively
  - local anesthetic infiltration plus acetaminophen. *Note:* patients with a history of snoring or sleep apnea may require continuous pulse oximetry monitoring postoperatively and smaller doses of morphine. The use of local anesthesia may allow the opioid to be omitted

- *Ventriculoperitoneal shunt:*
  - intraoperative intravenous opioid loading and local anesthetic infiltration by surgeon; postoperative i.v. opioid boluses or infusion, then oral codeine and acetaminophen as needed

- *Craniotomy:*
  - intraoperative acetaminophen loading plus i.v. opioid loading; postoperative i.v. opioid boluses as needed plus oral analgesia. Some patients will require opioid infusion or PCA

- *Frontoorbital advancement:*
  - intraoperative acetaminophen plus i.v. morphine loading; postoperative morphine infusion followed by oral analgesia, *or*
  - intraoperative morphine loading and postoperative PCA if suitable

- *Cleft palate surgery:*
  - Local anesthetic wound infiltration by surgeon plus acetaminophen loading and 0.1 mg/kg morphine; postoperative low-dose morphine infusion (up to 20 μg/kg per hour) or i.v. boluses as needed and acetaminophen

- *Squint repair:*
  - intraoperative acetaminophen loading plus topical local anesthesia if required; acetaminophen as needed postoperatively

16 Pediatric burns

Phil Gaukroger

Pain is experienced by all children with burns. In addition to the pain of the injury, children need to cope with the pain of debridement and surgical skin-grafting procedures and the need for frequent burn dressing changes. The pain is compounded by the devastating cosmetic and social effects of a burn injury not only on the child, but on the family as well. They are confronted with the prospect of permanent disability and disfigurement and future limitations in their daily activities.[1]

A 1982 survey[2] of US burn units showed that while adult burn patients had inadequate pain management, children were even more poorly managed. Since then, considerable improvements in pediatric acute pain management have resulted in more burns centers adopting improved methods for managing the considerable pain problems in children with burns. A 1994 survey[3] of analgesia regimens in 25 burns centers in the UK showed widespread use of·pharmacological techniques such as continuous opioid infusions (24 units), nitrous oxide and oxygen inhalation (16 units) and patient controlled analgesia (PCA) (4 units). Fourteen out of 19 units considered that assessment and control of pain are extremely difficult in children. Despite this progress, there is still scope for improvement in the control of pain in children with burns.

EPIDEMIOLOGY

Of all children with burns 52% are under 5 years old, 27% are aged 5–12 years, and the remaining 21% are 13–18 years old. More boys than girls sustain burn injuries. Infants and toddlers are most frequently scalded. Flame burns are more common in children older than 5 years.

Burn treatment

During the first few days following injury, medical efforts are aimed at resuscitation and survival with appropriate airway management, vigorous fluid replacement, prevention of sepsis, and management of pain. When the child becomes stable, surgical treatment of the burned areas begins.

In major burns with hypovolemia, redistribution of the circulation means that the cerebral and coronary circulations receive a relatively greater proportion of cardiac output while areas such as muscle and fat are poorly perfused. These patients are therefore more susceptible to the depressant effects of drugs such as morphine. Morphine should not be given intramuscularly (i.m.) or subcutaneously (s.c.) because initially it will not be absorbed from these sites. As fluid volume is restored, these depots will release the drug, and may cause delayed sedation or respiratory depression.

Opioids and sedatives given to these children during resuscitation should be given by small intravenous increments until the child is comfortable, and then analgesia can be maintained with a continuous intravenous infusion of morphine.

Burn dressing changes (BDCs) consist of removal of bandages, debridement of devitalized tissue, hydrotherapy, and application of antibacterial cream. Pain can be experienced during all these stages, particularly debridement. Many children become distressed and anxious and resist in a physical manner. Others may become catatonic, a state often described as 'learned helplessness'.

Debridement and skin-grafting procedures are performed under general anesthesia, often beginning 5–7 days following injury. Larger burns may require multiple procedures at intervals of a few days to a week. The donor areas constitute the source of greatest pain because normal skin is shaved. Nerve blocks (see Ch. 9) provide effective analgesia for donor areas such as the anterolateral thigh during surgery and in the initial postoperative period. Postoperative pain must be prevented from becoming severe, and having a child waking up comfortably in the recovery room is important in this respect.

After burns have healed, some children may have to return for surgical procedures such as contracture release, often years later. The procedures are usually straightforward, but these children are often extremely anxious due to vivid unpleasant memories of their previous hospitalization. This anxiety should be recognized and managed, often by allowing it to be expressed and by careful explanation of the procedures involved in this admission.

Many techniques of pain management – both pharmacological and nonpharmacological – are required for children with burn injuries. The techniques chosen will depend on the child's age, the child's ability to cope with hospitalization and the injury, and the preferences of staff in individual burns units.

Pain from burn injuries is often difficult to assess and control. Contrary to popular opinion, the magnitude of pain is proportional to the extent of burn injury. It is a myth that patients with third-degree burns do not experience significant pain. While nerve endings may be destroyed, areas of third-degree burns may have damaged nerve endings exposed giving rise to 'neuropathic pain' which is relatively resistant to opioids. The patient will also have other areas of lesser-degree burns which cause significant pain.

PHARMACOLOGICAL TECHNIQUES

Common pharmacological techniques for managing pediatric burn pain are outlined in Table 16.1.

Table 16.1 Pharmacological techniques for managing pediatric burn pain

Initial injury
- Titrate i.v. morphine to comfort
- Continuous infusion of morphine or consider starting patient-controlled analgesia (PCA) if patient suitable
- Add acetaminophen orally

Burn dressing changes
- Consider premedication with oral midazolam (especially in young patients)
- Nitrous oxide administration if suitable, *or*
- Intravenous sedation by anesthesiologist with appropriate monitoring and facilities (fentanyl/midazolam or ketamine/midazolam)
- General anesthesia for major cases

Postoperative pain following debridement
- Minor procedures: intravenous boluses of opioids followed by oral analgesics
- Major procedures: PCA if suitable. If unsuitable, continuous i.v. opioid infusion with nurse-administered boluses as needed. Oral analgesia with acetaminophen/codeine, or consider methadone or slow-release morphine if analgesia required for longer periods
- Nerve blocks covering donor areas for early postoperative analgesia

Simple analgesics

Simple analgesics such as acetaminophen (paracetamol) are widely used in burn units for the treatment of both minor pain and fever. In doses of 15–20 mg/kg acetaminophen is effective and free of adverse effects. In these long-term patients it is important not to exceed a dosage of 100 mg/kg per 24 hours because of the risk of hepatotoxicity.

The antiplatelet actions of nonsteroidal antiinflammatory drugs (NSAIDs) severely limit their use in children with burns, as any impairment to blood clotting can considerably increase blood loss during debridement and grafting procedures. These children are also stressed, and NSAIDs may increase the possibility of gastric erosions and bleeding from the upper gastrointestinal tract.

Opioid analgesics

Opioid analgesics continue to be the mainstay of analgesia for children with burn pain. As with other forms of acute pain, providing a suitable method of administration is of most importance in children. Intramuscular administration is intensely disliked by children and should not be used immediately after injury for the reasons outlined above. Intravenous and oral administration of these drugs is preferred.

Continuous intravenous opioid infusions (see Ch. 5) are commonly used to treat the pain of the initial injury and postoperatively. Most children with burn surface area greater than 10% will require intravenous access and are therefore easily managed initially with an intravenous morphine infusion.

Children should receive intravenous titration of small boluses (e.g. 20–40 μg/kg) of morphine until comfort is achieved. Their analgesia should be maintained with a variable infusion (usually up to 40 μg/kg per hour morphine) and ward nursing staff should be able to administer supplementary boluses of 30 μg/kg to cover incident pain. Children with major burns may develop acute tolerance to opioids. This is usually evident by the decreasing effectiveness of the opioid infusion, and can be managed by increasing the morphine infusion and bolus dose size and/or adding adjuvant drugs. If anxiety is considered to be a major component of the child's distress, then adding midazolam (at an initial hourly infusion rate of up to 40 µg/kg) to the infusion usually helps. The easiest way to achieve this is to add equal doses (in milligrams) of morphine and midazolam to the infusion. However, it must be remembered that this combination is potent and the child should be closely monitored for signs of oversedation. Amnesia from the midazolam is often a useful effect in these children.

Morphine remains the preferred opioid in children with burns. Meperidine's (pethidine's) metabolite, normeperidine, may cause neurotoxicity. Twitching and fits are the usual manifestations. Risk factors include higher doses, administration for more than a few days, and renal inpairment. Fentanyl is a useful alternative opioid for children sensitive to morphine side-effects such as pruritus and sedation. Fentanyl is unsuitable for routine use because acute tolerance develops very quickly.

Patient-controlled analgesia

Older children (usually over 7 years) can often be managed with PCA (see Ch. 6). This technique offers several benefits over staff-controlled opioid infusions. Children are able to control their pain relief to the level that they want, without having to ask for it or be continually assessed. This is particularly important in adolescents who desire control of their environment. Again, morphine is the preferred drug, and tolerance may develop. This is usually manifested by increasing demands from the PCA pump with inadequate analgesia. Tolerance is best managed by increasing the morphine concentration, bolus dose size and background infusion by 50%. Alternatively, if anxiety is significant or amnesia is desirable, then adding midazolam to the PCA machine will help to reduce the morphine requirements. A background infusion is normally given to patients with major burns, particularly if PCA is used for long periods. A background infusion in these children will contribute to better analgesia and also prevents the possibility of withdrawal effects in longer-term patients who are opioid-dependent.

The use of PCA has been described in children with burns for periods as long as 131 days.[4] In these children PCA was started at the time of first debridement although many centers now offer PCA soon after the initial injury. There was considerable variability in the morphine requirements of these children, and PCA allowed for wider ranges of doses than would normally be considered with opioid infusions. Three children developed tolerance to morphine, and this was easily managed by increasing doses. Children weaned themselves from opiates when skin closure was complete and painful procedures were no longer required. A pneumatic foot control was used in children with burnt arms who were unable to activate a PCA button normally. The use of PCA for long periods is possible where intravenous access is maintained with a long-term central venous catheter. In children with less serious burns, PCA can be used following debridement procedures and oral opioids used during the periods between debridements.

PROCEDURAL PAIN

There are a variety of techniques available to cover the pain of dressing changes. If i.v. access is available, titration with midazolam and fentanyl by an appropriately trained person in an area with full monitoring and resuscitation facilities can be used. Alternatively, if the child is on an opioid infusion or PCA, then a bolus (or several boluses if required) can be given prior to commencing the dressing.

Other agents have been used to alleviate the pain of BDCs. Ketamine is an anesthetic agent with profound analgesic properties. Its primary disadvantage is the occurrence of nightmares, which can be suppressed by benzodiazepines such as midazolam or diazepam. Although analgesic and sedative at low dosage, ketamine is a general anesthetic agent and even if used outside the operating room should usually be administered by an anesthesiologist with appropriate monitoring and resuscitation facilities.

With all sedation techniques for BDCs, it is essential that one staff member has responsibility for monitoring the child and maintaining verbal contact. Distraction techniques are a useful addition to this person's skills.

If intravenous access is not available, then inhalational analgesia with nitrous oxide (see Ch. 4) is a useful method for children capable of cooperating with its administration (Fig. 16.1). A protocol needs to be followed to avoid bone marrow toxicity from prolonged and repeated exposure. Some institutions limit nitrous oxide administration to no more than 1 hour per day and prescribe folinic acid to longer-term patients. The use of a mouthpiece for nitrous oxide administration is better accepted by children than a mask, and a mouthpiece is essential for children with facial burns (Fig. 16.1).

Oral premedication with midazolam 0.5 mg/kg (maximum 15 mg) 30 minutes before BDC has a reliable amnesic and anxiolytic effect which usually lasts 90–120 minutes. Oral midazolam is best suited to younger children requiring dressings. Its amnesic and anxiolytic properties improve the

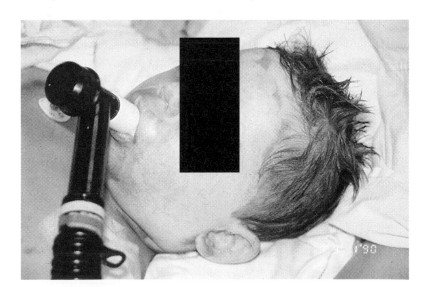

Fig. 16.1 Child with facial burns using mouthpiece for inhalation of nitrous oxide and oxygen during burn dressing change.

child's ability to cope with future procedures by preventing recollection of the previous procedure. Midazolam has no analgesic properties of its own and when used alone may not improve the child's acceptance of painful episodes. Coadministration of either nitrous oxide or an opioid are required for analgesia. Midazolam can also be administered intranasally (0.2–0.3 mg/kg). The advantage of this route is quicker onset, the disadvantage is that the solution may cause a burning sensation in the nose.

Oral opioids

Long-acting oral opioids such as sustained-release morphine or methadone (both with starting doses of 0.2 mg/kg 12-hourly) have become increasingly popular for children with burns because their use minimizes the duration of intravenous access and simplifies the method of administration, as twice daily dosing is usually adequate. Oral opioids such as these are useful for controlling background pain but are less effective in managing incident pain. Doses need to be titrated according to response. It may take several days for an increase in dosage to be effective, so administering an extra dose of methadone or short-acting oral morphine may be required. If a child has received these drugs for longer than 2 weeks, then the drug should not be stopped abruptly, but the dose should be decreased in stages to avoid the possibility of opioid withdrawal.

Prevention of pain-related problems is the best approach in children with burns. Pharmacological and psychological management should be used from the outset before difficulties arise and the patient becomes distressed.

NONPHARMACOLOGICAL TECHNIQUES

Nonpharmacological pain management techniques (see also Ch. 13) complement pharmacological techniques for these children and should be considered together rather than in isolation.

The room where BDCs are performed should be a relaxing environment, with distracting features on the walls and particularly on the ceilings. Suitable music playing continuously or perhaps the child's choice of radio stations helps to quell the quiet, cold atmosphere of a treatment room, and helps to relax the staff, who may be as distressed as the child during BDCs.

Giving the child control during painful episodes can reduce pain and distress. This can be done by giving the child some choices about the procedure and the opportunity to participate in the procedure. Control is an important element of the effectiveness of both PCA and nitrous oxide administration via a demand apparatus. These children frequently benefit from hypnosis and the entire spectrum of behavioral methods such as distraction, visual imagery and relaxation techniques.[5] A unit looking after children with burns should have staff trained in these techniques. Alternatively, an acute pain management service may be able to provide an appropriate person with these skills during BDCs.

Parental presence during procedures is controversial. Some units allow a parent to be present during distressing procedures to minimize separation anxiety and provide a distraction for the child.[6] This really is an issue which must be considered on an individual basis. The majority of children, particularly younger children, will prefer to have a parent or friend present. Parents, however, may become very upset by the procedure and find it difficult to be present. Some parents relax their child, while others may unwittingly make the procedure more distressing. Parents who wish to be present during these procedures need to be coached as to how they can best benefit their child. Techniques of distraction should be discussed beforehand. The parents need to be aware that their anxiety can be easily transferred to the child. They need to be fully aware of what is planned with each session.

FUTURE DEVELOPMENTS

Managing children with burns is one of the most difficult areas of pediatric pain management practice. There is considerable scope for improvement and pediatric acute pain management services should be encouraged to provide the expertise to manage the considerable procedural pain which occurs in the burns treatment room. We should aim for the humanitarian goal of having children experience as little pain as possible from their burn injuries.

REFERENCES

1. Carr DB, Osgood PF, Szyfelbein SK 1993 Treatment of pain in acutely burned children. In: Schechter NL, Berde CB, Yaster M (eds) Pain in infants, children and adolescents. Williams & Wilkins, Baltimore, pp. 495–504
2. Perry S, Heidrich G 1982 Management of pain during debridement: a survey of US burn units. Pain 13:267–280
3. Braam MJ, Bath AP, Spauwen PH, Bailie FB 1994 Survey of analgesia regimens in burns centres in the UK. Burns 20:360–362
4. Gaukroger PB, Chapman MJ, Davey RB 1991 Pain control in paediatric burns – the use of patient-controlled analgesia (PCA). Burns 17:396–399
5. Maron M, Bush JP 1991 Burn injury and treatment pain. In: Bush JP, Harkins SW (eds) Children in pain: clinical and research issues from a development perspective. Springer-Verlag, New York, pp. 275–295
6. George A, Hancock JJ 1993 Reducing pediatric burn pain with parent participation. Burn and Care Rehabilitation 14(1):104–107

17 Oncology

Meredith Gabriel

Considerable differences exist between children and adults in the nature of their cancers and the management of cancer pain (Table 17.1). Pediatric cancers are relatively uncommon; the majority are hematological (Table 17.2), and with aggressive therapy, most are potentially curable. Pain in children is therefore more commonly related to the therapy rather than to the tumor, as in adults.[1] The treatment of childhood cancer tends to be confined to specialist oncology units based in the larger pediatric hospitals. This chapter describes these differences as well as a number of practical aspects of the management of pain in children with cancer.

Table 17.1 Differences between pediatric and adult cancer

	Children	Adults
Incidence (% of all cancers)	Uncommon (1%)	Common (99%)
Tumour type	Mainly hematologic	Mostly solid tumours
Outcome	Mostly curable	Mostly incurable
Treatment	Very aggressive	Less aggressive
Pain problems	Therapy-related pain common	Tumor-related pain common
Palliative care	Usually short (weeks)	Often months to years
Bony metastases	Uncommon	Common
Managed by	Pediatric oncology team	Various specialities

Table 17.2 Incidence of pediatric malignancies

Tumor	Incidence (%)
Leukemias	30
Cerebral tumors	18
Lymphoma	13
Neuroblastoma	11
Wilms tumor	10
Bone tumors	5
Miscellaneous	13

EPIDEMIOLOGY

Tumor-related pain   The most common cause of tumor-related pain is the invasion of bone and bone marrow. Direct invasion of bone is commonly seen with osteosarcoma or Ewing's sarcoma, and bone marrow invasion occurs with leukemias and metastatic neuroblastoma. Bone pain is usually dull, aching, or boring. Involvement of several vertebral bodies causes paraspinal muscle spasm which results in sharp, excruciating pain. Rapid tumor growth or intra-tumor hemorrhage may cause severe, sharp pain. The exact constellation of symptoms will depend on the precise location of the tumor.

Soft-tissue tumors are more likely to be painless whether they are primary or metastatic. Pain ensues when there is local invasion of bone or nervous tissue, or obstruction of either a hollow viscus producing colic or a drainage pathway resulting in stasis and infection.

Headache is often the presenting symptom in children with brain tumors. Diffuse headache with vomiting may indicate raised intracranial pressure. Osteosarcoma and other soft-tissue sarcomas can metastasize to the brain parenchyma and cause diffuse headache also. Localized headache may be caused by cranial vault invasion, commonly due to neuroblastoma and Ewing's sarcoma. Less commonly, pain syndromes involving the base of the skull may be the presenting features of a tumor, the commonest being rhabdomyosarcoma.

Back pain has several etiologies. Spinal cord compression may cause localized, severe midline back pain, often exacerbated by coughing, straining, neck flexion, and straight leg raising. Paraspinal muscle spasm is commonly associated. Compression of the long tracts of the spinal cord and radicular pain may result in vague complaints of weakness, heaviness, or pain in the legs.

Pain caused by direct invasion of peripheral nerves is uncommon but can occur with chest wall tumors. Tumors invading the pleura can cause typical 'pleuritic' pain and either localized or radiating chest wall pain. Sometimes they are asymptomatic.

A small number of patients may have chronic pain persisting long after eradication of all tumor from the site of their pain.[1] These chronic pain syndromes may include phantom limb pain, persistent local pain following radiotherapy or systemic chemotherapy for sarcomas of bone or soft tissue, persistent headaches from cerebral irradiation, and neuropathic pain.

Therapy-related pain

The types of therapy undertaken depend on the tumor diagnosis and the stage at which it is diagnosed. Commonly, chemotherapy, radiotherapy, and surgery are used for primary or metastatic disease and for complications such as bowel obstruction. Therapy-related pain therefore encompasses blood tests, intravenous access procedures, investigations such as bone marrow aspirations and lumbar puncture, postoperative pain, infections, and other complications. Thus, the spectrum of therapy-related pain is wide.

The need for intravenous access for blood sampling, administration of chemotherapy and fluid therapy has been simplified by the insertion of long-term central venous catheters. These catheters have vastly reduced the number of needle insertions in these children and at the same time provide easy access for the administration of general anesthesia or intravenous sedation. These catheters can be either percutaneous (Broviac) catheters or completely implanted with a subcutaneous port. Accessing implanted catheters can still cause distress for some (particularly younger) children and the application of topical local anesthetic agent prior to access is useful.

Infection is a major cause of morbidity for cancer patients. It may be due to the malignancy itself or secondary to the immunosuppression caused by aggressive chemotherapy. Pain due to infection may be aching in nature as with systemic viral illness or septicemia, or more localized as in cellulitis, typhlitis, and perirectal cellulitis. Herpes zoster infection can occur in children but the associated pain is often transient, usually resolving over 1–2 weeks and seldom persisting beyond the resolution of the rash. It is usually localized, has a burning quality, and can be severe.

Mucositis is a common and very painful side-effect of chemotherapy or bone marrow transplantation. Generally, it is limited to the oral mucosa but can extend causing pharyngeal, esophageal and anorectal lesions. The pain of oral mucositis is difficult to control and local measures such as topical local anesthetics and mouthwashes have limited effect. Systemic opioids via patient-controlled analgesia (PCA) are usually required. Infections such as herpes simplex and candidiasis may also cause painful mucositis, and appropriate treatment should be instituted along with adequate analgesia.

Protracted vomiting and constipation secondary to chemotherapy may cause abdominal pain, but it is seldom severe. Occasionally gastritis may cause moderate to severe abdominal pain.

Radiotherapy may cause painful dermatitis and mucositis. Irradiation of paranasal sinuses, nasopharynx, and pelvis can be associated with severe pain. Abdominal irradiation can cause acute pain due to diarrhea. Radiation-induced nerve damage is uncommon but the neuropathy caused by chemotherapy or direct tissue injury by tumor may be exacerbated.

Neuropathic pain can occur in children with cancer. The three main causes are surgical interruption of nerves causing phantom limb pain, chemotherapy, and radiotherapy. Tumor invasion of nerves or a major nerve plexus is less common. Drug-induced peripheral neuropathy is mainly caused by vincristine and has a dysesthetic, burning quality. It is mostly experienced by teenagers. Younger children seldom complain of dysesthetic pain.

Headache after lumbar puncture is uncommon in children and is more likely to occur in adolescents than in younger children. It is exacerbated by sitting or standing and relieved by lying down. The headache usually resolves with time, but an epidural blood patch may be required for persistent cases.

EVALUATION OF CANCER PAIN IN CHILDREN

Evaluation of cancer pain should include:

- The quality and intensity of pain
- The precise location of the pain
- The etiology of the pain
- The estimated duration of the pain

- The analgesic history
- The child's ability and preferences with regard to medications and their route of administration

Parents have an important role in the assessment and management of pain in children with cancer. Parents give useful information about the child's ways of expressing pain and anxiety, especially where the child is too young to talk. Involving parents closely with the management of painful procedures and treatment may help to allay their own anxiety and enables them to help their child deal with the many new and difficult situations that they have to face.

MANAGEMENT OF CANCER PAIN IN CHILDREN

Treatment methods can be pharmacological, psychological, and physical, and it is usually a combination of all three which is most effective. Which modalities are chosen depend on the cause of the pain, the age and coping abilities of the child, and the facilities available. The best available methods should be used at the start of treatment and not be reserved for cases where difficulties arise. Pain should be anticipated and treated preemptively. Painful procedures should be planned and combined to minimize the number of episodes of intervention. The initial treatment of the tumor often relieves pain simply by reducing tumor cell mass. Generally some other form of pharmacological analgesia will be required while waiting for tumor shrinkage or recovery from surgery.

Pharmacological methods

Analgesics are most often given orally or intravenously as these routes are most acceptable to children. The majority of these children have implanted central venous catheters making intravenous administration simple. Intramuscular administration is disliked by children and may cause major bruising when thrombocytopenia is present. Rectal administration is usually avoided in immunosuppressed children owing to the risk of bacteremia. The subcutaneous route is usually disliked because it involves a needle insertion and children have to carry a small infusion pump; however, it is a useful route during the later phases of palliative care.

Table 17.3 outlines options and dosages of the commonly used analgesics in pediatric oncology.

Simple analgesics

Acetaminophen (paracetamol) is the most common first-line analgesic drug used in these children as it is nonsedating, relatively free from side-effects, and very useful for less severe pain. Nonsteroidal antiinflammatory drugs (NSAIDs) are rarely used except for bone pain and in palliative care. They are avoided due to their antiplatelet effects and gastric irritation, both undesirable in oncology patients. Simple analgesic drugs are discussed in Chapter 3.

Opioids

Opioid analgesics such as codeine, morphine, methadone, oxycodone, and fentanyl are the mainstay of pain management in children with cancer.

Table 17.3   Analgesic dosage guidelines in pediatric oncology

Drug	Prescription	Comments
Acetaminophen	15–20 mg/kg orally every 4 hours 25–30 mg/kg rectally every 6 hours	For mild pain, antipyretic
Naproxen	5–7 mg/kg orally every 12 hours	Available as syrup, tablets, suppositories
Ketorolac	1 mg/kg loading dose then 0.5 mg/kg i.v. or s.c. every 12 hours	Parenteral NSAID
Codeine	0.5–1 mg/kg orally every 4 hours	Partial opioid agonist

Morphine	0.1 mg/kg i.v. bolus every 1–2 hours as needed
	0–50 μg/kg per hour i.v. or s.c. infusion
	PCA:
	  bolus 15–20 μg/kg
	  background 15 μg/kg per hour	

Methadone	0.2 mg/kg i.v. bolus 0.2 mg/kg orally ever 12 hours	Oral starting dose
Fentanyl	1–3 mg/kg per hour i.v. infusion	Short-acting drug, alternative to morphine
Midazolam	0.5–0.75 mg/kg oral dose at once or 0.05–0.2 mg/kg i.v. up to 0.5 mg/kg 0–100 mg/kg per hour i.v. or s.c. infusion	Premedication or for sedation
Amitriptyline	0.5–1.5 mg/kg at bedtime	Low doses usually adequate for co-analgesic effect Higher doses for treatment of depression
Doxepin	0.2–2 mg/kg orally every 8 hours	Maximum 100 mg/dose
Dexamethasone	0.1 mg/kg orally or i.v. daily	

Codeine has been extensively used as it is well tolerated orally, both alone or in combination with other simple analgesics such as acetaminophen. Unwanted effects such as nausea and constipation as well as a dosage ceiling limit the extent to which codeine is useful.

Morphine and to a lesser extent methadone are the most commonly used drugs when simple analgesics are inadequate for the control of pain. Side-effects such as nausea, vomiting, and pruritus may limit dose escalation. Morphine is the most common drug used with PCA and opioid infusions (see Chs 5 and 6).

An increasing number of oral morphine preparations are now available. In the past morphine was simply available as a syrup which was relatively short-acting and unpalatable. The slow-release preparations now available as tablets or 'sprinkles' are much more acceptable because they are easy to take and require only twice daily dosing. A dose of 0.2 mg/kg 12-hourly is a common starting dose and the drug is subsequently titrated to effect. Requirements vary considerably between individuals. Escalation of dosage is usually required in palliative care and parents need to know that this is normally the case.

Opioids are not ideal analgesics for bone pain and the addition of an NSAID such as naproxen can markedly improve the quality of analgesia in children with bone pain.

Oral methadone was commonly used before the introduction of slow-release morphine preparations as it is a drug with a long half-life requiring only 12-hourly administration in most children. The starting dose is 0.2 mg/kg 12-hourly and it is then titrated to effect.[2] Methadone is available in a syrup which may make it suitable for children who are unable to take slow-release morphine.

Oxycodone is a short-acting opioid which is available as tablets or suppositories It can be used as an alternative to codeine as an oral analgesic or can be administered rectally when effects such as vomiting limit the usefulness of oral preparations.

Fentanyl is primarily used as a short-acting intravenous analgesic for painful procedures. Transdermal fentanyl patches have been approved in some countries for the management of cancer pain, and are simple to apply and well accepted by patients. They take 12–24 hours to have an effect after application, and can take a similar time to wear off after discontinuation.

Local anesthetic agents

Local anesthetic creams are commonly used for venipuncture, for insertion of intravenous or subcutaneous cannulae, for accessing subcutaneous ports, and for other minor procedures such as lumbar puncture. A little forward planning such as the parent applying local anesthetic cream at home prior to coming to hospital can make a significant difference to the performance and perception of the many painful procedures a child with cancer has to face.

Regional techniques such as epidural blockade may be used for postoperative pain but are rarely used in pediatric palliative care. The main reason for this is that pediatric cancers are unlikely to produce the types of pain that are suitable for epidural techniques. Bony metastases, which are the most common indication for epidural techniques in adult palliative care, are uncommon in pediatric oncology.

Corticosteroids

Corticosteroids are indicated for treatment of pain secondary to raised intracranial pressure from a cerebral tumor, spinal cord compression, nerve plexus compression, and tumor-related peripheral nerve compression. They may also be useful for treatment of widespread metastatic bone pain. Their mechanism of action is presumably reduction of local edema. Dexamethasone is usually the drug of choice because it has the highest penetration into the central nervous system. It is also useful for the management of nausea secondary to chemotherapy or during palliative care.

Adjuvant drugs

The tricyclic antidepressants (TCA), amitriptyline and doxepin, are useful in treating the depression experienced by patients with life-threatening illnesses and also deafferentation pain. They have a synergistic effect with other analgesic drugs as well. Patients often find that sleep improves immediately and pain is reduced within 4–5 days. If a child with cancer pain requires night-time sedation, starting a TCA is often a better option than benzodiazepines because of their co-analgesic effects.

Midazolam (see Ch. 3) is a short-acting benzodiazepine commonly used for its amnesic properties during painful procedures; it may also be useful for anxiety and agitation, especially the restlessness that can occur in the terminal phase. It can be administered intravenously, subcutaneously, orally, or transmucosally, making it an extremely versatile and useful drug in pediatric oncology.

Specific antiemetics, in particular ondansetron, are indicated for nausea and vomiting related to chemotherapy or general anesthesia.

Antiepileptics such as carbamazepine or phenytoin can be beneficial for neuropathic pain when antidepressants are not effective.

POTENTIAL PROBLEMS SPECIFICALLY RELATED TO PEDIATRIC CANCERS

Immunosuppression   Children with cancer are intrinsically immunosuppressed as well as having iatrogenic immunosuppression related to their chemotherapy. Consequently, vigilance must be maintained for subtle signs of infection, especially if simple analgesics are being used for the management of the child's pain. Both acetaminophen and the NSAIDs have potent antipyretic properties and can mask the onset of fever related to infection. Careful monitoring of opioid analgesic therapy is also needed, because an intercurrent illness such as severe infection or the administration of chemotherapy may suddenly alter the susceptibility of the child to the effects of the opioid and a rapid alteration in dose may be required.

Thrombocytopenia   Another consequence of chemotherapy and sometimes of the primary disease is thrombocytopenia. A tendency to bleeding limits the use of NSAIDs. This tendency as well as susceptibility to infection also limits the use of the rectal route for drug administration.

Prolonged use of opioids   Addiction is of concern to some parents when their child is commenced on long-term opioids. It must be explained to them that children do not become 'addicted' to opioids; however, they will develop some physical dependence so that if these drugs are no longer required, they should be withdrawn slowly and not abruptly stopped. Physical dependence will occur if the child requires opioids for a period of several weeks or longer, so that once pain is no longer a problem, slow reduction over 1–2 weeks is necessary because a withdrawal reaction may occur if the drug is ceased abruptly. Withdrawal symptoms include jitteriness, sweating, and irritability.

Tolerance develops with prolonged use of opioids. It can be managed either by adding co-analgesics such as NSAIDs, tricyclic antidepressants, midazolam or low-dose ketamine, or increasing morphine dosage. There is no upper limit to the dose of morphine that can be prescribed. Some children receiving palliative care can require as much as several grams of morphine a day.

NONPHARMACOLOGIC TECHNIQUES

Nonpharmacologic methods (see also Ch. 13) help children to cope with both the pain and their cancer. These methods are best used in combination with pharmacological approaches and can reduce the requirements for drugs and improve analgesia.[3]

In pediatric oncology a clinical psychologist is often involved, although all staff should be familiar with the simpler techniques. Hypnotherapy, distraction techniques, positive feedback, giving control to the child, play therapy, and relaxation therapy are all ways of controlling pain without drugs and will improve the analgesia obtained from pharmacological techniques.

Physical methods of pain relief play a role in the overall management of cancer pain and include massage, application of heat and cold and transcutaneous electrical nerve stimulation (TENS). Transcutaneous electrical nerve stimulation can be used for a variety of pain problems, generally of a more chronic nature, such as phantom limb pain.

TECHNIQUES FOR PROCEDURAL PAIN

General anesthesia

Bone marrow biopsies and lumbar punctures are a major pain management problem in pediatric oncology. General anesthesia administered by specialist anesthesiologists in appropriately equipped and monitored areas is routinely used in many units, especially for younger children. With careful planning, other procedures such as intravenous therapy or blood sampling can be done painlessly at the same time.

Conscious sedation

Conscious sedation refers to the administration of intravenous analgesics, amnesics or sedatives to achieve a state where the child is still conscious and able to respond, but usually has no recollection of the procedure. It is routinely used in many centers for bone marrow biopsies and lumbar punctures, and is an acceptable alternative for the child who does not like general anesthesia for these procedures.

Conscious sedation is commonly achieved by intravenous titration of midazolam and fentanyl, which achieves the desirable combination of amnesia and analgesia, and as these drugs are short-acting, recovery is relatively quick. Midazolam and fentanyl can be a very potent combination, however, with potential for respiratory depression and respiratory arrest, particularly in sick cancer patients. It is essential that guidelines and protocols be established for this technique, that continuous pulse oximetry be used, that full resuscitation facilities are available and that an appropriately trained person is solely responsible for the patient's wellbeing. Other drugs such as ketamine have been used, but may contribute to a slower recovery and hallucinations.

Nitrous oxide inhalation

The use of nitrous oxide (see Ch. 4) for short procedures such as lumbar punctures is simple and easy and has the benefits of rapid onset, rapid recovery, and no need for intravenous access.

Hypnotherapy

Hypnotherapy (see also Ch. 13) can be of considerable benefit for school-aged children. It is especially useful for procedural pain in cancer patients because they have regular invasive procedures over a long course of treatment and review, allowing time for them to master the technique.

PALLIATIVE CARE

Although survival rates are increasing for most pediatric cancers, children die from their disease and in these cases will benefit from palliative care.[4,5] Unlike adults, most children have a relatively short terminal phase lasting a few weeks to 2–3 months. The main focus of palliative care is to ensure that the child is comfortable, enjoys life as much as possible, and is able to die peacefully. Parents need extra support during this time. The decision to stop active treatment with the aim of cure or at least remission can be devastating to them.

Home care or institutional care?

Where to manage the dying child depends on the wishes of the child, the family, and the extent of support facilities available. In the majority of cases, palliative care can be carried out at home, which in most cases concurs with the wishes of the child. Hospice care is available in some centers. Few children elect to have palliative care in the acute care hospital setting, but it may be necessary if their condition has suddenly deteriorated or their imminent death has been precipitated by complications of therapy.

Therapy must be individualized to the needs of each child. Excellent support services for home care are often available from community nursing services. In addition, the family doctor is often involved, especially as this person will have an important role in the continuing care of the family after the child dies. Some children are able to attend school until very near their death. In these cases, the school staff and students will need to be counseled appropriately.

Pain management

The methods discussed above for the management of acute pain should all be available for the care of the dying child. Some children have very little pain and can be managed with oral analgesia until very late in their illness. Other children, often with neuroblastoma or sarcomas, have more severe pain which escalates rapidly.

Discussion about pain management should occur very soon after the decision to abandon active therapy has been made. Most parents dread the thought that their child might suffer severe pain. Parents will need advice on what to expect, and on methods of controlling symptoms such as vomiting and constipation as well as analgesia.

As the cancer progresses, the pharmacokinetics and pharmacodynamics of analgesic drugs may alter. Gut absorption of drugs can diminish owing to gastrointestinal stasis and edema. Dysphagia may develop in some cases. Progressive drowsiness may make oral administration of drugs difficult. In these cases, alternative routes of administration – rectal, subcutaneous, or intravenous – need to be considered.

Although analgesics are the mainstay of pain relief, palliative chemotherapy may play a part in the relief of symptoms.

Pharmacological options

A progression of therapies similar to the World Health Organization 'analgesic ladder' is adopted by most clinicians experienced in this area.

The first step is to use simple analgesics such as acetaminophen, or acetaminophen and codeine mixtures. If bone pain is significant, NSAIDs such as naproxen are available in syrup, capsule and suppository formulations and are used instead. Tricyclic antidepressants are used if pain is neuropathic or if inadequate sleep is a problem.

Children who have significant pain despite receiving simple analgesics are usually started on regular long-acting oral opioids such as slow-release morphine or methadone. Some slow-release morphine preparations can be given as 'sprinkles' mixed in with the child's favourite food, making administration easier. If necessary NSAIDs and tricyclic antidepressants are added as co-analgesics. Meperidine (pethidine) does not have a place in palliative care because of accumulation of the neurotoxic metabolite normeperidine. Oral oxycodone tablets or morphine syrup can be given as a supplement for breakthrough pain. The majority of children can be managed for all or most of their palliative care with oral analgesia.

If the oral route is not tolerated or has become ineffective despite escalating dosage, then an alternative route of administration will need to be considered. Many pediatric oncology patients still have the option of intravenous access available to them via a permanent central venous catheter. This route is well accepted if available, and a morphine or morphine/midazolam infusion can be administered by an ambulatory or bedside pump depending on the child's mobility. If the child is also taking an oral NSAID, then it may be worthwhile changing this to intravenous ketorolac if bone pain remains. Patients on intravenous morphine infusions should have the facility for bolus doses to cover incident pain. In some children, PCA is their preferred option in palliative care, and with ambulatory PCA devices now available, home PCA is a viable alternative. A background infusion is necessary when prescribing PCA for palliative care and should cater for at least half the child's daily morphine consumption.

If intravenous administration is not available, subcutaneous infusions are the most commonly used option. These are usually administered via a small ambulatory pump, usually with the contents of a syringe being administered over 24 hours. A subcutaneous butterfly needle is inserted after application of local anesthetic cream, and the site is usually able to tolerate up to 0.5 ml per hour without puffiness. The site is changed when required, and may last from 1 day to 2 weeks between changes. Subcutaneous infusions are usually only required when children are no longer ambulant.

Midazolam can be added to both intravenous and subcutaneous morphine infusions where sleeplessness, restlessness, agitation, seizures, or muscle spasm are a problem. Usually 1–2 mg/kg is added to the syringe to be administered over 24 hours; however, there are considerable differences between individual children and titration to effect is necessary.

Dexamethasone is often used to reduce tumour edema and control nausea. Hyoscine or atropine can be administered to control oral secretions which tend to pool in the oropharynx and cause distressing symptoms in the last few days of life.

CONCLUSION

With a multimodal approach to the management of pain experienced by the child with cancer, both the illness and its aggressive treatment can be made more tolerable. Infants and children have special needs, and pain management techniques must be tailored to these needs and not simply be scaled-down adult techniques. The needs of parents and the broader family must be taken into account. Caring for dying children requires the skillful use of all treatment modalities so that the children are capable of enjoying life to the end with minimal pain and side-effects. Prevention of the development of chronic pain syndromes is paramount if the survivor of childhood cancer is to have quality life thereafter. The importance of adequately managing pain of all etiologies and at all stages of care cannot be overemphasized.

REFERENCES

1. Miser AW, Dothage JA, Wesley RA, Miser JS, 1987 The prevalence of pain in a pediatric and young adult cancer population. Pain 29:73–83
2. Fainsinger R, Schoeller T, Bruera E 1993 Methadone in the management of cancer pain: a review. Pain 52:137–147
3. McGrath PJ, Finley GA, Turner CJ 1994 Making cancer less painful – a handbook for parents. Oncology Unit, Izaak Walton Killam Children's Hospital and Dalhousie University, Halifax, Nova Scotia.
4. Kohler JA, Radford M 1985 Terminal care for children dying of cancer: quantity and quality of life. British Medical Journal 291:115–116
5. Oakhill A 1988 Terminal care. In: Wright J (ed.) The supportive care of the child with cancer. Butterworth, Oxford, pp 243–259

18 Pain relief in the newborn

Peter Loughnan, Jag Ahluwalia

INTRODUCTION

Can newborn infants feel pain? In the past, many of those caring for newborns in hospital believed that their patients were unable to feel pain, and that even if they could, infants would not remember it.[1] These views were based on a belief that the neural pathways involved in nociception were 'immature' at birth. It was also observed that infants' behavioral responses to various stimuli seemed erratic and inconsistent. These beliefs and observations led some physicians to ignore the issue of analgesia in the newborn, and led to widespread practices which would now be regarded as inhumane.[1] In recent years, the neurophysiology of pain in the newborn has received considerable attention. Pain receptor density in newborn skin is similar to that of adults. The central connections of these receptors are nearly complete by about 30 weeks of gestation. Nociceptive stimuli can be carried in unmyelinated or thinly myelinated nerve fibres.[2] The neuropeptides, monoamines and catecholamines which are implicated in pain pathways in adults are present in fetal life. In summary, the basic connections of the pain pathways are present at birth, but some components of this system continue to develop postnatally. As stated by Fitzgerald, 'the human neonate undoubtedly has the neuronal apparatus to detect painful stimuli, but perhaps in a less organised way than the human adult'.[3]

PAIN ASSESSMENT

The assessment of pain in the newborn is difficult. An infant's response to a range of stimuli, noxious and otherwise, is limited. Taking a heel-prick blood sample may elicit the same changes in facial expression, heart rate, and body posture as undressing the infant for examination. Consequently the assessment of pain, and in particular its severity, cannot be an exact science. The corollary to this is that assessment of the effectiveness of analgesia may also be difficult. Nevertheless, a number of approaches have been used by different authors in an attempt to develop reliable and accurate tools with which to measure pain in the neonate.[4]

Pain assessment in the newborn is based on observing changes in various markers associated with painful experiences. As there is no subjective report available from the infant and pain is a subjective experience, these measures are necessarily indirect. The following areas have been used to provide measures of neonatal pain:

● Biochemical and metabolic changes
● Behavioral changes
● Physiological changes

Pain is associated with altered levels of various catecholamines as well as glucagon, insulin, endogenous corticosteroids, and biochemical markers for protein catabolism.[5] Several behavioral scoring systems have been described, usually involving a semiquantitative score assigned to features such as facial expression, body posture, withdrawal response, muscle tone, and restlessness. These summate to a pain score.[6] Certain physiological parameters are also altered by pain, including heart rate, blood pressure, and cutaneous blood flow. Such methodologies are primarily used in research studies, and in the evaluation of the efficacy of different analgesic regimens.

While biochemical and metabolic changes may provide the most reproducible measurement of the response to pain, in practice the use of behavioral and physiological changes is likely to remain the basis for pain assessment in routine clinical care. Behavioral observations and even the interpretation of physiological parameters are imprecise, and can be influenced by factors other than pain. Gestational age and the infant's behavioral state are important in this respect. However, experienced neonatal nurses will be applying a 'pain score', consciously or unconsciously, to each infant in their care. The nurse's clinical assessment should be carefully considered by the physician responsible for pain relief.

Certain pitfalls in pain assessment should be borne in mind. While pain is often associated with restless or agitated behavior, on occasions some infants with severe pain will remain almost completely immobile. The use of muscle relaxants in ventilated infants decreases our ability to assess their pain. Therefore it is inevitable that on occasions our assessment of pain can be difficult or even impossible. When this occurs it is suggested that a physician's choice of analgesia may be more appropriate if the question is asked: 'What form of pain relief would I request if I were subjected to this procedure or circumstance?'.

WHY TREAT PAIN?

Any discussion of treating pain in an infant needs to consider not only the side-effects of the treatment but also the advantages and disadvantages of pain perception. With the exception of providing signs which assist in the evaluation of an ongoing pathological process, such as abdominal tenderness with peritonitis, the presence of pain in the newborn would appear to confer few, if any, biological advantages. In contrast, an infant's perception of pain seems to result in a number of physiological (and possibly psychological) disadvantages.

The infant's response to pain results in a number of potentially adverse physiological changes. Cardiovascular responses include elevations in heart rate, blood pressure, and intracranial pressure, as well as falls in oxygenation. In the sick preterm infant such fluctuations are known to be associated with an increased incidence of intraventricular hemorrhage and necrotizing enterocolitis. Adverse sequelae also arise from the stress response associated with pain. The release of glucagon, catecholamines, and endogenous corticosteroids leads to a catabolic state and is associated with an increased incidence of postoperative complications.[7] Other body systems are involved in the response to pain including the immune and hemostatic systems. For example, infants whose pain response is ameliorated during and after surgery have a reduced incidence of postoperative thrombotic complications and disseminated intravascular coagulation.[7] The experience of pain in the neonatal period may decrease pain sensitivity later in childhood.[8]

In summary, there would appear to be considerable data supporting the view that pain offers the sick infant few advantages, and that its treatment improves both the short-term and long-term outcome. These factors are superimposed upon the ethical position that we should not allow infants to suffer avoidable severe pain.

NONPHARMACOLOGICAL PAIN MANAGEMENT

A number of nonpharmacological strategies can be used to minimize the effects of pain in the newborn infant. Such strategies are listed in Box 18.1 and discussed below. Often they will be used in conjunction with drug therapy.

Box 18.1. Adjuncts to drugs in neonatal pain management

- Relief of precipitating events
- Comforting
- Feeding
- Oral sucrose
- Refrigerant sprays
- Reduction of environmental noxious stimuli

Mechanical causes of pain may require a mechanical solution. For example, splinting of a painful limb lesion, or the relief of abdominal distension with a nasogastric tube, may be all the analgesia that is required. For infants distressed by poor synchrony with a ventilator, the careful use of patient-triggered ventilation may obviate the need for pharmacological analgesia or sedation. This also may produce an improvement in gas exchange, whereas opioid analgesia in the same circumstance can result in respiratory depression and prolong the course of ventilator dependence.

The simple act of comforting, for example by nursing the infant in its mother's arms, or by oral feeding when this is clinically appropriate, may provide sufficient modulation of the painful process such that drugs are no longer required. Nonnutritive sucking during painful procedures such as heel-prick sampling has a pacifying effect. Oral sucrose reduces the level of distress and apparent pain in infants undergoing brief painful procedures. The release of endogenous endorphins in response to oral sucrose is a postulated mechanism for this observation. Refrigerant sprays may be used to decrease the pain associated with intramuscular injections in young infants. Stimulation of nonpain-associated afferent sensory pathways can inhibit pain perception (see Ch. 13). The beneficial effect of cuddling or stroking an infant may in part utilize this mechanism.

The distress caused to infants in neonatal intensive care can be minimized by careful coordination of painful procedures, and by minimizing unpleasant environmental stimuli. For example, in an infant with peritonitis, routine nursing procedures such as turning and diaper changing can be timed to coincide with the physician's palpation of the abdomen. The elimination of unnecessary noise, lighting and other potentially distressing stimuli may produce beneficial short-term changes in physiological parameters, and long-term benefits in recovery from disease, and weight gain.[9] Thus an integrated approach to pain management that includes nonpharmacological modalities may have a significant impact on both the degree of pain perception by an infant, as well as upon the requirement for pharmacologically mediated analgesia.

DRUG TREATMENT OF PAIN IN THE NEWBORN

The choice of an analgesic should take into account both the reason for requiring analgesia and the underlying disease state. For example, short-lived pain from a minor procedure in a nonventilated infant should not be treated with drugs that may produce significant respiratory depression. On the other hand, postoperative analgesia for an abdominal surgical procedure in a ventilated preterm infant with severe hyaline membrane disease may be given with less regard to its effects on spontaneous respiration. The choice of analgesic may be restricted by the infant's ability to tolerate enteral drug administration. There is no ideal analgesic agent. The selection of drug will depend on the severity of pain, the infant's general medical condition, and the drug's adverse effects.

Systemic analgesic drugs

Opioids

Opioid analgesics such as morphine, fentanyl, diamorphine, and sufentanil are available for the treatment of newborn infants with severe pain. Meperidine (pethidine) is not commonly used in the newborn. Morphine is the most widely used opioid in newborn nurseries, and there are more data available regarding its pharmacokinetic properties than for the other drugs. There seems little to choose between the various opioid analgesics. All have similar central nervous system depressant effects at equianalgesic doses. Because of its widespread usage in the newborn, morphine is discussed here in further detail.

Morphine has both analgesic and sedative effects. In neonatal intensive care units, this drug is usually given as a continuous intravenous infusion, but it can also be administered orally, intramuscularly, or by intermittent intravenous bolus. Rapid intravenous bolus doses should not be used in the newborn as they cause acute respiratory depression and hypotension. Loading doses may be required and should be administered by infusion over at least 30 minutes. Oral absorption of morphine in adults is incomplete and variable. This has not been studied in the newborn. The onset of morphine's action is somewhat delayed, owing to its slow penetration into the central nervous system because of its relatively low lipid solubility. This effect may be lessened by the immature blood–brain barrier and the rapid circulation in neonates.

In adults morphine is eliminated mainly by hepatic conjugation to morphine 3- and 6-glucuronides which are then excreted in the urine. Morphine 6-glucuronide is a pharmacologically active opioid agonist. The production of morphine 6-glucuronide is greatly impaired in the newborn. The low levels of this active metabolite could explain the high plasma concentrations of morphine required for analgesia in the newborn[10] (see below).

The mean half-life of morphine is 6–8 hours in the first week of life, longer in those who are critically ill, and is about 10 hours in preterm infants. This compares with a half-life of approximately 2 hours in adults. It is important to note that, as with many hepatically metabolized drugs, the half-life of morphine in the newborn is highly variable. It is inevitable that the use of fixed infusion rates will produce widely different plasma morphine concentrations and therefore pharmacological effects in different babies. Owing to this variability a dose likely to be effective and well tolerated must be selected and titrated to need. The authors' practice is to use a continuous infusion of 20–25 μg/kg per hour in ventilated infants, but a lower dose of 10–15 μg/kg per hour is used in those breathing spontaneously. An infusion rate of 20 μg/kg per hour produces adequate analgesia in most infants[11] and mean steady state morphine concentrations of about 100 ng/ml. This compares to levels of about 65 ng/ml required for analgesia in older children.[11] This requirement for higher morphine plasma concentrations in the newborn is unexpected but possibly explained by the low levels of the active metabolite morphine 6-glucuronide produced by newborns.[10] These morphine levels can produce respiratory depression. A loading dose of 50–100 μg/kg over 30 minutes may be necessary in infants with severe pain, as the full effect of a continuous infusion is not obtained for several hours. The above doses may be exceeded in ventilated infants with severe pain, according to clinical response. Morphine infusions in ventilated infants should usually be stopped, or reduced to less than 15 μg/kg per hour for at least 12–24 hours, before anticipated extubation.

Excessive plasma concentrations of morphine have been associated with central nervous system depression, gastrointestinal immotility, and urinary retention. These adverse effects are reversible. Seizures were reported in two critically ill infants in an early study using relatively low-dose morphine infusions.[12] The authors have not observed this problem, and seizures have not occurred in several subsequent studies using higher-dose infusions. Hypotension due to peripheral vasodilatation is rarely seen in the newborn except with rapidly administered loading doses. For this reason hypovolemia should be corrected before commencing morphine infusions.

Benzodiazepines

An alternative approach to opioid administration in ventilated infants who require sedation rather than analgesia is midazolam, a relatively short-acting benzodiazepine, given as a continuous infusion of 20–60 μg/kg per hour.[13] The combination of a benzodiazepine and an opioid enables the use of lower doses of opioid in adults and children. Although this combination seems logical and has been used for neonates requiring sedation and analgesia, its place in the treatment of the newborn is not established. There are potential problems with tolerance and withdrawal with these regimens.

Acetaminophen

Acetaminophen (paracetamol) is safe and effective in infants with moderate pain judged not to require opioid administration.[14] It is metabolized primarily by hepatic conjugation to both glucuronide and sulfate. The sulfate conjugate predominates in the newborn. A small fraction of the drug is oxidized by the hepatic cytochrome P450 system to a highly reactive arene compound which is inactivated by glutathione conjugation. It is this arene metabolite which causes hepatic necrosis following acute acetaminophen poisoning in adults. The cytochrome P450 pathway is considerably slower in the fetus and newborn, thus newborn infants may be protected against this serious adverse effect of excessive plasma acetaminophen concentrations. This, combined with the lack of reports of hepatic toxicity in the newborn, would indicate that fear of hepatotoxicity should not unduly limit the use of this drug in the newborn.[14] Acetaminophen is well absorbed orally in newborn infants, although peak concentrations are somewhat delayed compared to adults. The plasma half-life is about 4 hours, compared with 2 hours in adults and older infants. Oral acetaminophen can be given on a regular 6-hourly basis in a dose of 15–20 mg/kg. It can also be administered rectally, but absorption is incomplete and variable. Rectal doses of 25–30 mg/kg can be used 8-hourly. Exact doses are limited by available suppository formulations. Irrespective of route, a maximum daily dose of 100 mg/kg should not be exceeded. There is little information regarding the pharmacokinetics of acetaminophen in premature infants. General principles would suggest that lower doses or a longer dosage interval would be appropriate in the preterm patient. Acetaminophen is safe and effective in the newborn, can reduce the requirement for opioid analgesia, can be given rectally and does not require intravenous access for administration. This drug is underutilized in neonatal practice.

Other systemic analgesic drugs

Oral opioid drugs, such as morphine and codeine, and the nonsteroidal antiinflammatory drugs could be useful analgesics in the newborn, but there is little published information regarding their use. In particular, oral opioids combined with appropriate sedation should be considered during the palliative care of infants without venous access. Acetaminophen often proves inadequate in these situations. Ketamine is another drug that may have a role in providing analgesia in selected infants.[15]

Local anesthetic drugs

Local anesthetic agents have a large role in pain relief and prevention in neonates undergoing surgery or invasive procedures. The safety, profound analgesia, lack of sedation, and long duration of action of single injections of bupivacaine with added epinephrine (adrenaline) make this an almost ideal analgesic technique. This is especially true for neonates who often require analgesia for a shorter duration postoperatively. For inguinal hernia surgery, a single perioperative bupivacaine injection, by caudal epidural, ilioinguinal field block or surgical infiltration, may be the only analgesia required.

Safe use of local anesthetic drugs in neonates requires appropriate training, resuscitation facilities, and an understanding of the differences between the pharmacology of these drugs in neonates compared with older children and adults.

Apart from prilocaine (see below), toxic levels of local anesthetic drugs in neonates appear to be similar to those in adults.[16] On a per kilogram basis, maximum single doses of bupivacaine and lidocaine for blocks are the same as for adults. Where local vasoconstriction is not contraindicated, epinephrine 5 µg/ml can be added to the local anesthetic solution to decrease peak blood levels and increase the safety margin of higher doses. The keys to avoiding acute toxicity are careful calculation of the maximum dose and avoidance of intravascular injection. Low doses delivered intravascularly may cause convulsions or cardiac arrest.

A 2-fold to 3-fold increase in the volume of distribution (per kg), of bupivacaine in neonates compared with adults, combined with a similar clearance (per kg), means that the elimination half-life of bupivacaine in neonates is 2–3 times that of adults.[17] This is relevant to repeat injections or infusion techniques. The authors do not use more than 0.25 mg/kg per hour for postoperative epidural infusions in neonates and usually stop the infusion by 24 hours. This is usually sufficient duration for profound analgesia in neonates and decreases the risk of toxicity, because blood levels of bupivacaine may continue to rise over 2–3 days and, although the dose is low, toxic levels could occasionally be reached with infusions of this duration.

Lidocaine (lignocaine) has similar changes in pharmacokinetics compared with adults as bupivacaine, but its short duration of action means that prolonged analgesia will not be achieved with a single injection. It seems that lidocaine may be more prone to tachyphylaxis than bupivacaine when used for epidural infusions. These shortcomings tend to restrict the use of lidocaine, which is suitable when rapid onset of local anesthesia is required for procedures not expected to cause much postoperative pain. It may be used topically in the airway.

Mepivacaine has a very low clearance in neonates due to their poor ability to perform aryl hydroxylation. The volume of distribution is 2–3 times greater than that of adults (per kg), so the elimination half-life of mepivacaine is very long in neonates.[18] Given the availability of alternative drugs, there seems little indication for mepivacaine in neonates.

Prilocaine should be avoided in the newborn because it is particularly prone to cause methemoglobinemia in neonates.[19] About 80% of neonatal hemoglobin is fetal, which is more easily oxidized to methemoglobin than adult hemoglobin. Neonatal red cells are more prone to hemolysis due to reductive agents, so ascorbic acid is recommended for the treatment of methemoglobinemia in neonates rather than methylene blue.[20]

CONCLUSION

Newborns do feel pain. Unless that pain is transient, it should be ameliorated where possible. There will probably never be an ideal analgesic, but sufficient information is available to enable adequate relief of pain using both pharmacological and nonpharmacological approaches. The provision of adequate analgesia in the newborn with severe pain requires intensive monitoring, available in modern neonatal intensive care units. Pain relief results in benefits such as a reduction of postoperative complications and shortened hospital stay; nevertheless, the humanitarian goal of relieving the infant's pain remains paramount.

REFERENCES

1. Gauntlett IS 1987 Analgesia in the newborn. British Journal of Hospital Medicine 37:518–519
2. Colditz P 1991 Management of pain in the newborn infant. Journal of Paediatrics and Child Health 27:11–15
3. Fitzgerald M 1993 Development of pain pathways and mechanisms. In: Anand KJS, McGrath PJ (eds) Pain in neonates. Elsevier Science, Amsterdam, pp 19–37
4. Fitzgerald M, McIntosh N 1989 Pain and analgesia in the newborn. Archives of Disease in Childhood 64:441–443
5. Anand KJS, Sippell WG, Aynsley-Green A 1987 Randomised trial of fentanyl anaesthesia in preterm babies undergoing surgery: effects on the stress response. Lancet i:243–248
6. Taddio A, Nullman I, Koren BS, Stevens B, Koren G 1995 A revised measure of acute pain in infants. Journal of Pain and Symptom Management 10:456–463
7. Anand KJS, Hickey PR 1992 Pain and stress responses in neonatal cardiac surgery. New England Journal of Medicine 326:1–9
8. Grunau RV, Whitfield MF, Petrie JH 1994 Pain sensitivity and temperament in extremely low birthweight premature toddlers and preterm and fullterm controls. Pain 58:341–346
9. Mann NP, Haddow R, Stokes L, Goodley S, Rutter N 1986 Effect of night and day on preterm infants in a newborn nursery: randomised trial. British Medical Journal 293:1265–1267
10. Chay PCW, Duffy B, Walker J 1992 Pharmacokinetic-pharmacodynamic relationships of morphine in neonates. Clinical Pharmacology and Therapeutics 51:334–342
11. Levene MI, Quinn M 1992 Use of sedatives and muscle relaxants in newborn babies receiving mechanical ventilation. Archives of Disease in Childhood 67:870–873.
12. Koren G, Butt W, Chinyanga H, Soldin S, Yok-Kwang T, Pape K 1985 Postoperative morphine infusion in newborn infants: assessment of disposition characteristics and safety. Journal of Pediatrics 107:963–967
13. Jacqz-Aigrain E, Daoud P, Burtin P, Desplanques L, Beaufils F 1994 Placebo-controlled trial of midazolam sedation in mechanically ventilated newborn babies. Lancet 344:646–650
14. Anand KJS, Shapiro BS, Berde CB 1993 Pharmacotherapy with systemic analgesics. In: Anand JKS, McGrath PJ (eds) Pain in neonates. Elsevier Science, Amsterdam pp 155–198
15. Hartvig P, Larsson E, Joachimsson P 1993 Post operative analgesia and sedation following pediatric cardiac surgery using a constant infusion of ketamine. Journal of Cardiothoracic and Vascular Anesthesia 7:148–153

16. Brown TCK, Fisk GC 1992 Paediatric anaesthetic pharmacology. In: Brown TCK, Fisk GC (eds) Anaesthesia for children, 2nd edn. Blackwell, Oxford Ch 2, pp 44–46
17. Bricker S, Telford R, Booker P 1989 Pharmacokinetics of bupivacaine following intercostal nerve block in neonates and infants less than 6 months. Anesthesiology 79:942
18 Moore RG, Thomas J, Triggs DB et al 1978 Pharmacokinetics and metabolism of anilide anaesthetics in neonates. European Journal of Clinical Pharmacology 14:203
19. Mandel S 1989 Methemoglobinaemia following circumcision. Journal of the American Medical Association 261:702
20. Menahem S 1988 Neonatal cyanosis, methemoglobinaemia and haemolytic anaemia. Acta Anaesthesiologica Scandinavia 77:755

19 Management of pain in pediatric intensive care

Robert Henning

INTRODUCTION

Critically ill children often suffer pain which may be difficult to detect and assess. The attention of staff is often concentrated on treating the child's illness, and the sick child's pain may be overlooked. The autonomic signs of pain are often attributed to other causes such as heart failure, shock, or sepsis. Assessment of pain is also made difficult by problems with communication. Adequate analgesia in the critically ill child is not only humane but can prevent the responses to pain which stress the child's limited reserves and confuse diagnosis. Satisfactory pain relief may also speed recovery by increasing mobility and preventing the adverse psychological effects of unrelieved pain. Details of the pain management of neonates in intensive care are discussed in Chapter 18.

THE PATIENT

Children of all ages may require intensive care. They may be unable to communicate their pain because of their developmental stage (Ch. 2), the severity of their illness, particularly central nervous system effects, and treatments such as sedatives, muscle relaxants or artificial ventilation. Assessment of pain in these closely monitored patients, especially infants and paralyzed children, depends on autonomic responses such as tachycardia, hypertension, and sweating, and the response to simple comforting measures and to analgesic drugs. This may even apply to older children who have previously communicated well but who may regress to earlier developmental stages or become withdrawn in response to critical illness and intensive therapy. Other factors such as fear, guilt, embarrassment and absence of a parent may exacerbate pain and inhibit communication in toddlers and older children.

Many teenagers and older children who are treated in intensive care units after major elective surgery (e.g. cardiac or spinal surgery) can use the same pain management methods as other postoperative patients of the same age, including patient-controlled analgesia (PCA), although in the first few hours after operation this may not be feasible. In most critically ill children and teenagers, confusion, disorientation and sedation prevent the use of pain control methods which depend on patient cooperation or reliable communication.

THE ILLNESS

The sources of pain will vary with the illness and treatment. Analgesia should be tailored to the circumstances. Pain after spinal surgery in a teenager needs substantial analgesia for some days, while pain due to an intercostal catheter may be relieved by removing the catheter.

The nature, severity, and complications of the child's illness may also affect the pharmacokinetics and pharmacodynamics of analgesic drugs. Critically ill children frequently have impaired function of multiple organ systems. Renal and hepatic dysfunction are common in children with septic shock, multiple trauma, or burns and after open heart surgery (especially in infants, those with critically low aortic blood flow before operation, and babies after deep hypothermic circulatory arrest), prolonging the action of drugs excreted by the liver or kidneys. In these conditions, hypoalbuminemia often alters the plasma protein binding of drugs.

Capillary leak of protein-laden fluid, paralytic ileus and the subsequent fluid resuscitation increase the volume of distribution of drugs. The loading dose of a drug needed to achieve therapeutic concentrations is therefore increased, but continuing drug requirements are decreased owing to impaired renal and hepatic clearance (in drugs eliminated by these routes). The elimination half-life is prolonged by decreased clearance and by the increased volume of distribution. Impaired gut blood flow in the severely ill often precludes enteric administration of analgesic drugs, or makes enteral bioavailability unpredictable. Intramuscular injections are rarely indicated in the critically ill because of variable muscle blood flow and because of associated coagulopathies.

Children with painful conditions requiring prolonged intensive therapy often develop increasing requirements for analgesic and sedative drugs owing to acute tolerance. Rapid reduction of dose may be complicated by withdrawal phenomena. This is rare in children treated with opioids for less than 5 days, but becomes increasingly common as the duration and total dose of opioid therapy increases. Newborn babies treated with extracorporeal membrane oxygenation (ECMO) and sedated with fentanyl infusions, augmented if necessary with benzodiazepines, commonly show signs of opioid withdrawal if the fentanyl is given for longer than 5 days or the total dose exceeds 1.6 mg/kg.[1] Signs of opioid abstinence syndrome seen in pediatric intensive care unit (PICU) patients include excessive crying, tremors, fits and myoclonic jerks, increased muscle tone, frequent yawning, sweating, salivation, sneezing and nasal stuffiness, tachypnea, vomiting, frequent watery stools, fever, shortened sleep periods, and excessive sucking. These symptoms impair recovery, nutrition, and weight gain, and slow the resumption of spontaneous breathing. Withdrawal symptoms should be anticipated in infants and children at high risk and prevented by slow reduction of opioid dose, combined with the use of other sedatives such as benzodiazepines. In the setting of withdrawal from several days of high-dose opioid therapy, the presence of several of the signs of abstinence syndrome should arouse suspicion, but the signs are nonspecific and other complications, such as sepsis, pneumonia, or cardiac failure, should be excluded.

SOURCES OF PAIN

Wounds, fractures, and indwelling tubes and catheters often cause pain in children in intensive care. Pain may also be caused by procedures, immobility or by the underlying condition (e.g. muscle pain in Guillain–Barré syndrome).

Children with conditions that are usually painful should receive appropriate doses of analgesic drugs even if their distress cannot be detected directly owing to their condition or treatment, such as in the presence of head injury or muscle relaxants. Movement that could be expected to exacerbate pain should be preceded by analgesia. For example, extra analgesia is usually needed before chest physiotherapy in children after thoracotomy or before turning a child after spinal surgery. Continuous analgesia is needed in the first few days in children with chest wounds to minimize the pain due to breathing and to permit coughing.

Indwelling catheters are responsible for much of the misery suffered by children in PICU. Intravenous catheters are often painful, especially in the presence of phlebitis or if irritant drugs are injected through them. Peripheral intravenous sites should be observed frequently and changed if phlebitis occurs. Irritant drugs should be avoided or administered through central veins. Analgesic drugs in conventional doses are not usually effective in preventing pain due to phlebitis or the injection of irritant drugs. Similarly, the discomfort of nasogastric and endotracheal tubes, and of intercostal, urinary, and peritoneal catheters, is difficult to abolish with usual doses of analgesic drugs, especially if the discomfort is made worse by movement, coughing, or other frequently occurring events.

Many ICU procedures are painful,[2] including tracheal suction, turning, physiotherapy, and removal of stitches, catheters, endotracheal tubes, or pacing wires. Children with fractures or the muscle pain of Guillain–Barré syndrome often fear mobilization, including passive limb movement, which causes severe pain. These repeated painful treatments, combined with helplessness, immobility, enforced bed rest, difficulty in communication, and prolonged hospitalization, contribute to the depression and withdrawal which is often seen in children with Guillain–Barré syndrome. The pain of planned but infrequently occurring procedures such as the removal of catheters or drains may be reduced by the prior administration of drugs such as opioids or ketamine, combined with discussion with the child and a kind, gentle approach on the part of the carer. For frequently repeated painful maneuvres such as tracheal suction and the fluid inflow phase of peritoneal dialysis, intermittent premedication with analgesics may not be practical, short of opioid drug infusion. Unless the child needs an opioid infusion for another reason, the best method of minimizing the child's distress from these procedures is explanation and use of a gentle technique.

In older children and teenagers, mobilization is often inhibited by wound pain or its anticipation. Analgesia sufficient to reduce the pain without impairing the ability to cooperate should be given prior to the planned movement. Immobility may cause pain, especially in older children, due to muscle cramps and the need to rely on passive positioning by PICU staff. Staff should avoid both overstretching the child's joint capsules and ligaments by maintaining the joints in the position of function, and excess or prolonged pressure on skin or bony prominences from the bed or hard objects including splints and catheters.

FACTORS THAT INCREASE PAIN PERCEPTION

The severity of the pain suffered by a child from a given painful stimulus is affected by endogenous factors as well as by the child's surroundings. Critically ill children are often confused because of their illness, sedation, sleep deprivation or an altered pattern of sleep, steroid administration, noise, unfamiliarity with their surroundings, and the absence of their parents and familiar objects. This reduces their ability to cope with painful stimuli, increasing the distress associated with a particular stimulus.

Pain perception is also affected by a child's morale. A cheerful, optimistic child is likely to interpret a given stimulus as less painful than a child demoralized by prolonged hospitalization, recurrent painful procedures, worries over prognosis, or by depression or guilt (e.g. fantasies that the illness may be punishment for some real or imagined fault of the child). Anxious or angry parents who may themselves feel guilty over the child's illness readily communicate this anxiety to their child, amplifying pain perception. Parents and children of different cultural backgrounds have different ideas of how much pain should be expected from different painful stimuli, and how that pain should be dealt with. A stoical child may suffer severe pain which may only be discovered by direct questioning. Appropriate analgesia should be given, despite the stoicism.

Although it is difficult in the short term to influence factors such as depression, guilt, anxiety, or cultural expectations which may be amplifying the child's perception of pain, arrangements for the child to be cared for by a small group of nurses and doctors whom the child and family trust, rather than by the larger group of all PICU staff as dictated by the vagaries of the roster, may help lessen the anxiety. Discussions with the child and family about pain and analgesia (as well as about other aspects of the child's care) can improve the child's morale and help the family to best support the child, reducing the pain experience. These discussions require considerable tact and insight on the part of staff into the situation and views of each family, and must be true discussions and not merely lectures from staff to parents.

THE EFFECTS OF PAIN

Pain has evolved at least in part as a warning system. Although pain may provide useful diagnostic information, in the PICU most effects of pain are negative. Relief of pain is not only humane but can prevent many complications. Pain inhibits movement, so adequate analgesia, especially after thoracic and abdominal surgery, can facilitate mobilization. This decreases atelectasis and nosocomial pneumonia, reduces the risk of deep venous thrombosis in teenagers (DVT is rare in young children), and accelerates the resumption of normal bowel function and the resorption of edema fluid when capillary leak syndromes have occurred.

Pain increases the intracranial pressure and the cerebral metabolic rate, and adequate analgesia with opioids is an essential part of the management of acutely raised intracranial pressure, provided that the child is appropriately ventilated to prevent hypoventilation and hypercarbia. Mechanical ventilation may be indicated in multiple trauma with only moderate head injury in order that adequate analgesia can be safely provided without the risk of hypercarbia raising the intracranial pressure.

In systemic hypertension (e.g. after coarctation of the aorta repair or liver transplantation) and pulmonary hypertension (e.g. after cardiac surgery), adequate analgesia can improve pressure control and minimize antihypertensive requirements by preventing pain-induced, sympathetically mediated increases in vascular resistance. High-dose opioid analgesia has been essential in management of infants with persistent pulmonary hypertension of the newborn or pulmonary hypertension after cardiac surgery, although since the introduction of nitric oxide therapy, it has not been necessary to use the same anesthetic doses of fentanyl or morphine as previously.

The stress response to injury and severe illness involves the release of catecholamines, glucocorticoid and neuropeptide hormones, as well as cytokines such as tumor necrosis factor (TNFα), interleukin 1 and interleukin 6, causing fever and increased resting energy expenditure (including increased oxygen consumption and carbon dioxide production). Catabolism of fat and protein is increased, while increased gluconeogenesis and reduced hepatic uptake of glucose due to insulin resistance produce hyperglycemia. There is also retention of sodium and water. This stress response is amplified by pain, and although its magnitude and duration can be reduced by the administration of local anesthetic or anesthetic doses of opioids,[3] it is not affected (in adults) by conventional doses of opioids sufficient to give adequate analgesia.[4] Although there is a suggestion that outcome may be improved by suppression of the stress response,[5] the evidence is not conclusive. The costs of complete suppression of the stress response include the side-effects of high-dose opioids, and prolongation of intubation and mechanical ventilation. It is not clear that the stress response is wholly maladaptive or that its suppression is likely to benefit critically ill children.

In sick, semiconscious children, pain contributes to distress and disorientation, and pain relief often makes such children much more rational and cooperative.

PAIN VERSUS AWARENESS IN PICU PATIENTS

Ideally, a child in the PICU should be alert, cooperative, and pain-free. However, distress may arise from psychological and physical sources other than pain. For example, inability to move, communicate, or avoid noxious stimuli because of pharmacological paralysis can be highly unpleasant although painless.[2] Opioids, even in high dose, do not reliably produce unconsciousness or amnesia. The combination of an analgesic dose of opioid with a sedative often provides better pharmacological relief of distress than escalating doses of opioid alone. The anxiolytic, amnesic properties of benzodiazepines are useful for this purpose. Good general care includes talking to the child and around the bedside as if the child were aware. Simple measures such as warning the child before performing any procedures, noxious or otherwise, telling the child who you are, what time it is, and what is happening, and generally making occasional conversation appropriate to the child's age may greatly reassure apparently unaware children. *Staff should take care to limit bedside conversations with other staff and parents to what they would want the child to hear.*

Control of agitation by sedation, not necessarily including analgesics, may be important in some patients. In severe tracheobronchomalacia, agitation greatly increases expiratory airway obstruction. Sedation with minimum impairment of respiratory drive, for example with a benzodiazepine combined with a phenothiazine or butyrophenone titrated against the child's conscious state and respiratory pattern, may facilitate successful weaning from mechanical ventilation. The addition of an opioid may be needed to reduce the pain of tracheal suction, although at the expense of reduced respiratory drive.

ASSESSMENT OF PAIN

Awake, nonintubated, older children of normal intelligence can describe their pain and factors that exacerbate or relieve it, and can tell you if analgesia is adequate. Children in intensive care, however, are often too young or too shy to give this information.

Tracheal intubation prevents vocalization. Lip-reading may help in older children, but not all staff or families are sufficiently skilled. A pen and paper, or a communication board on which the alert, intubated, older child or carer can point to boxes that say 'pain', 'itchy', 'nose', 'arm', 'drink' etc., may be useful. Self-reporting scales of pain severity may be useful guides to pain management, although most children remain in the PICU for too short a time to learn to use the scales effectively. For most PICU patients, staff estimate the severity of the child's pain by observing pain behavior or physiological responses to pain. Pain behavior includes crying (spontaneously or in response to maneuvers such as turning or limb movement), grimacing, avoidance of movement, or drawing up the legs.

In paralyzed children and very young infants, physiological changes are the most reliable indicators of pain, for example tachycardia, hypertension, pupillary dilation, sweating and skin vasoconstriction, and the response of these variables to painful stimuli and to analgesic drugs. All of these physiological variables are often abnormal in critically ill children (especially those with shock, heart failure, sepsis, or hypovolemia), and experience is needed to assess the role of pain in producing a particular pattern. For example, acute hypertension, especially if associated with other signs such as pupillary dilatation in a critically ill child, is much more likely to be due to pain than to other causes such as heart failure, provided seizures, intracranial hypertension, and hypercarbia can be excluded.

Children with severe heart failure (e.g. after open heart surgery) may not be capable of raising their blood pressure above normal, and pain may only produce tachycardia, sweating, and pupillary dilatation. In a child with a denervated heart after heart transplantation, pain causes little increase in heart rate, and may not increase the blood pressure, so sweating, pallor, and dilated pupils may be the only signs of pain, and their appearance should lead to examination of the child, and a trial bolus of an analgesic drug after other causes of these phenomena such as hypercarbia, hypovolemia, and a full bladder have been excluded.

NONPHARMACOLOGICAL METHODS OF PAIN MANAGEMENT

Any obvious avoidable sources of pain should be managed or removed. These may include joints in an abnormal posture, pressure on the skin from splints, painful skin sutures, intravenous cannulae, or decubitus ulcers. Pain caused by peritoneal dialysis or intercostal catheters may be relieved by repositioning the catheter or the child. Nonpharmacological methods of pain relief are described in Chapter 13.

When painful procedures are unavoidable, they should be kept to a minimum, and the child should be told beforehand exactly what is going to happen and why. This should also be done with paralyzed children who cannot give a sign that they understand what is being said to them, and with toddlers who appear too young to understand. One should never say: 'This won't hurt', if the procedure is obviously going to hurt, but rather, 'This will hurt, but only for a moment and then I'll get you a drink' (for example). Painful procedures and the reasons for them should also be discussed beforehand with the child's parents (if present), so that their anxiety over the child's suffering does not amplify the child's own anxiety and pain. If the parents seem likely to remain calm during the procedure, their presence may greatly reduce the child's distress, but the presence of anxious, excitable parents during procedures is likely to increase the child's distress.

Other measures include feeding the child and promoting sleep, conversing gently with the child, keeping the child warm and comfortable, making the surroundings as nonthreatening as possible, and encouraging the child's parents to be with the child as much as is compatible with their own rest, nutrition, and good humor. Sometimes the promise of a 'reward' after a procedure may reduce its unpleasantness. Rewards may include sips of fluid, a dressing with a smiling face or cartoon figure, reading a story, games, television, etc. Although children in pain find it very difficult to concentrate on the usual forms of entertainment, they may be more receptive after the pain is relieved by analgesics, and entertainment may help avoid the demoralizing effect of boredom.

FACTORS AFFECTING THE CHOICE OF ANALGESIC METHOD AND DOSE

Some aspects of intensive care management (e.g. disorientation, enforced immobility, tracheal intubation, and colic due to constipation) are extremely unpleasant, but are better relieved by methods other than using analgesic drugs. The site of the pain and the age of the child affect the usefulness of nerve blockade. The prospect of repeated intercostal nerve blocks may be acceptable to a teenager who understands that they may only be needed once or twice, but not to a 5-year-old who imagines this torture going on forever. For injuries in which adequate analgesia may require blockade of several nerves over a long period, an alternative technique such as local anesthetic infusion blocks or intravenous infusion of an opioid is usually preferable.

The child's underlying condition or its complications often affect the choice of analgesic technique. Major local anesthetic techniques are contraindicated in a child with significant coagulopathy. If the coagulopathy can be corrected transiently and there is a strong indication (e.g. caudal epidural block has been used to restore skin blood flow in meningococcal septic shock), these techniques may be used. Spinal or epidural anesthesia is not appropriate in the presence of known or suspected raised intracranial pressure of any cause. Spinal or epidural local anesthesia is relatively contraindicated in any child with a decreased ability to increase cardiac output (such as those with aortic or mitral stenosis, hypoplastic aortic arch, coarctation of the aorta, pericardial effusion, or a cardiomyopathy). Whether the heart is capable of maintaining an adequate blood pressure despite loss of vascular tone, as will occur with the sympathetic blockade caused by epidural or spinal anesthesia, can be tested by giving a carefully monitored trial infusion of a short-acting vasodilator such as sodium nitroprusside. The use of spinal or epidural anesthesia is best avoided in the presence of septicemia, although it is not an absolute contraindication.

In a child with barely adequate respiratory or myocardial function, especially during the phase of weaning from respiratory or inotropic drug support, the dose and choice of analgesic drug used is often a compromise between the need to provide adequate analgesia and the need to avoid opioid-induced hypotension and hypoventilation. This requires close monitoring of the child's breathing and circulation and frequent adjustments to the drug infusion rate. Excessive doses of opioids will prolong the need for mechanical ventilation, with its risks of sepsis, air leak, atelectasis, nosocomial pneumonia and accidental extubation, and may decrease cardiac output and blood pressure and increase the requirement for inotropes.

As discussed above, the presence of renal or liver impairment, capillary leak, and hypoproteinemia affects the pharmacokinetics of analgesic drugs and therefore the size of a loading dose and the rate of infusion needed to give adequate analgesia. The sedative and analgesic effects of an opioid infusion may last 48 hours or more after the infusion is stopped in a patient with poor drug elimination. This should be taken into account when planning a child's weaning from mechanical ventilation. The infusion should be withdrawn or tapered off in anticipation of decreasing requirements. Renal impairment is a contraindication to meperidine (pethidine) use owing to the risk of normeperidine toxicity.

PHARMACOLOGICAL APPROACHES TO ANALGESIA

The main options for drug treatment of pain in critically ill children are:

- Local anesthetic techniques, including topical anesthesia, nerve blocks, and spinal or epidural blocks
- Nonsteroidal antiinflammatory drugs (NSAIDs) and acetaminophen (paracetamol)
- Opioid drugs with or without adjuvants such as phenothiazines or benzodiazepines
- Systemic anesthetic agents which may be used in low dose for sedation and (in some cases) analgesia or as general anesthesia for procedures.

Although nitrous oxide inhalation is used for procedural pain and isoflurane has been used for long-term sedation, inhalational analgesic techniques are not commonly used in PICUs. Ketamine has profound analgesic effects at low dose, and at high dose is a general anesthetic with a unique mechanism of action. Propofol, a short-acting intravenous anesthetic agent, has been used for procedural pain, but infusions for sedation have been associated with metabolic acidosis and death in critically ill children.

Local anesthesia

Topical anesthesia, local infiltration, or nerve blocks should be used to abolish the pain of wounds, fractures, procedures such as insertion of venous or arterial cannulae, urinary catheters, intercostal or peritoneal dialysis catheters or endotracheal tubes, or manipulation of fractured limbs. This is especially true for paralyzed children and even for those who are receiving opioid infusions which may be insufficient to abolish the acute pain of procedures. Topical anesthesia of the airway should precede awake tracheal intubation, or intubation of a child with raised intracranial pressure.

Epidural blockade (see Ch. 7) can be used after thoracotomy including after cardiac surgery. For open heart surgery, where full heparinization is used and postoperative coagulopathy is common, epidural blockade is not advised because of the risk of epidural hematoma.

Although normal children under about 8 years old are not sensitive to the sympathetic blockade of epidural block, many children in PICU rely on sympathetic drive to maintain their cardiac output and blood pressure, or cannot increase cardiac output to maintain blood pressure in response to venous pooling and decreased systemic resistance caused by sympathetic blockade. Therefore epidural blockade is usually contraindicated in children who have poor myocardial function, cardiac valve stenosis or large residual aortopulmonary shunts (e.g. due to collateral vessels in tetralogy of Fallot or pulmonary atresia), or in whom cardiac output is limited by hypovolemia, pericardial effusion, or septicemia.

Acetaminophen and NSAIDs

Acetaminophen or NSAIDs, sometimes combined with codeine, may provide sufficient analgesia in some PICU patients (see also Ch. 3).

Combinations of acetaminophen and codeine are useful in nonventilated children with head injury or after craniotomy.

Nonsteroidal antiinflammatory drugs should be avoided in children who are prone to gastric bleeding (e.g. those with raised intracranial pressure, burns, shock, coagulopathy, treated with glucocorticoids, or receiving no enteral feeds); NSAID-induced nephrotoxicity is more common in children with preexisting renal impairment, heart failure, or hypovolemia, and in those on nephrotoxic drugs such as aminoglycosides, frusemide, or amphotericin.[6] These drugs should also be avoided when inhibition of platelet function is hazardous (e.g. in children with intracranial bleeding or cerebral infarction, and in those with coagulopathy due to liver failure).

Opioids and adjuvants

Infusion or intermittent bolus administration of opioid drugs (see Ch. 5) is the mainstay of pain control in critically ill children. The cardiovascular, respiratory, central nervous system, and gastrointestinal effects of opioids are especially likely to be clinically significant in PICU patients.

An intravenous morphine bolus can cause marked vasodilation owing to histamine release and reduction of sympathetic tone, and so is especially likely to produce significant cardiovascular depression in children with reduced cardiovascular reserve. Boluses of fentanyl and sufentanil reduce ventricular systolic performance less than morphine but more than alfentanil. This effect is greater in infants in severe heart failure whose cardiac output and blood pressure are dependent on the child's own sympathetic tone, and is less in children on high-dose infusions of inotropic drugs. If a bolus of an opioid is needed in a hypotensive child or one whose myocardial function is poor, alfentanil or fentanyl are preferable to morphine. Morphine infusions do not usually affect the circulation and can be safely used even when the child's cardiac output is profoundly reduced. Alfentanil reduces ventricular diastolic compliance, and could exacerbate conditions associated with ventricular hypertrophy, especially obstructive hypertrophy.

Gastrointestinal side-effects of opioids seen in critically ill children include gastric stasis and paralytic ileus which increase the risk of vomiting, regurgitation and aspiration, and reduce the ability of the child to tolerate enteral feeding. This ileus may be so severe and prolonged that parenteral feeding, with its attendant risks, is required to maintain the child's nutritional state. In general, however, enteral feeding can continue via a nasojejunal tube despite heavy sedation with opioids and administration of muscle relaxants.

Opioids (especially fentanyl and its derivatives) in high dose may rarely cause seizures,[7] particularly in newborns. High-dose opioids should be used with caution if seizures have been difficult to control, especially if muscle relaxants impede the monitoring of seizures. Sedation due to opioids can contribute to the disorientation which is common in all intensive care patients. Patient-controlled analgesia (Ch. 6) is an ideal method of delivering opioids to relatively alert older children or teenagers (for example after cardiac or other major surgery), but most PICU patients are too young or too ill to make use of such devices.

When tolerance to opioids is becoming troublesome, addition of a small intravenous dose of a phenothiazine such as chlorpromazine or a butyrophenone such as haloperidol may allow lower doses of opioid to be used, at the expense of a little extra drowsiness, or may provide better analgesia than was achievable with the opioid alone. Both of these groups of drugs may cause hypotension when given by intravenous bolus. They should be given slowly or in small increments, and the blood pressure monitored. When they are given for short periods at low doses for these restricted indications, the incidence of complications such as dystonic reactions, tardive dyskinesia and neuroleptic malignant syndrome is extremely low.

Benzodiazepines provide sedation, anxiolysis, and amnesia, which can relieve distress and lessen the pain experience of the child. Rapid intravenous boluses may cause marked respiratory and cardiovascular depression. Doses of midazolam as low as 40 μg/kg followed by an infusion of 1–4 μg/kg per minute may be effective, especially as a supplement to an opioid infusion. Acute tolerance to benzodiazepines may occur. If high doses are used for long periods, sudden cessation of the drug may cause acute withdrawal which may be associated with seizures. This is more likely with short-acting agents without active metabolites, such as midazolam. The short duration of action and lack of active metabolites of midazolam are usually an advantage as they allow rapid titration of the effect.

Anesthetic agents

Ketamine

The hypnotic and profoundly analgesic effects of ketamine are used in severely ill children especially before painful procedures, and to take advantage of the indirect sympathomimetic effects of the drug. Ketamine is widely used in the PICU before such procedures as burns dressings, bone marrow puncture, and insertion of intercostal drains. It is also used in asthmatic children as a bolus before tracheal intubation and as an infusion during mechanical ventilation, to take advantage of its mild bronchodilator action. In hypotensive children, the sympathetic stimulation caused by ketamine usually maintains a normal or slightly increased blood pressure despite the direct myocardial depressant effect of the drug. In children whose blood pressure is already dependent on a maximal endogenous sympathetic drive, ketamine may markedly reduce the blood pressure. Ketamine can worsen pulmonary hypertension,[8] although there is doubt that this occurs in children. It seems prudent to avoid ketamine in children with pulmonary hypertension, as alternative sedative, anesthetic and analgesic agents are available.

Ketamine increases the cerebral metabolic rate and raises the intracranial pressure, and should be avoided in children with intracranial hypertension. It also lowers the seizure threshold in children who are prone to seizures. Benzodiazepines, and to a lesser degree opioids, can minimize emergence phenomena, nightmares and hallucinations due to ketamine. The usual anesthetic induction dose of ketamine is 1–2 mg/kg i.v., which may be followed by an infusion of 0.5–2 mg/kg per hour (8–33 μg/kg per minute). For analgesia, doses as low as 5 μg/kg per minute may be effective. Ketamine can cause bronchorrhea and sialorrhea. Antisialogogues should be given if needed, not routinely.

Nitrous oxide

Nitrous oxide (N_2O) has a rapid onset and offset of analgesia and is easy to administer (see also Ch. 4). It is useful for reducing the pain of brief procedures in the PICU, where it should be administered by personnel trained in anesthesia, with appropriate equipment and scavenging. Some of the problems that limit the use of nitrous oxide are more common in the PICU than in the rest of the hospital. Significant closed, gas-containing cavities which can be expanded (or pressurized) by nitrous oxide include pneumothoraces, unventilated gas-containing lung segments, and obstructed paranasal sinuses and middle ear cavities (which are common in children undergoing prolonged nasotracheal intubation). Many critically ill children have abnormal immune function and poor nutrition, and a need for repeated procedures that may otherwise be suitable for nitrous oxide analgesia. These are just the circumstances where the adverse effects of nitrous oxide on bone marrow and leukocyte function could become manifest, excluding many patients from this therapy. Nitrous oxide should be avoided in children with impaired myocardial function and in those with pulmonary hypertension, as it may exacerbate both conditions.

REFERENCES

1. Arnold JH, Truog RD, Orav EJ, Scavone JM, Hershenson MB 1990 Tolerance and dependence in neonates sedated with fentanyl during extracorporeal membrane oxygenation. Anesthesiology 73:1136–1140
2. Hayden WR 1994 Life and near-death in the intensive care unit. A personal experience. Critical Care Clinics 10(4):651–657
3. Anand KJ, Sippell WG, Aynsley-Green A 1987 Randomised trial of fentanyl anaesthesia in preterm babies undergoing surgery: effects on the stress response. Lancet i:62–66
4. Møller IW, Dinesen K, Søndergård S, Knigge U, Kehlet H 1988 Effect of patient-controlled analgesia on plasma catecholamine, cortisol and glucose concentrations after cholecystectomy. British Journal of Anaesthesia 61:160–164
5. Anand KJS, Hickey PR 1992 Halothane-morphine compared with high-dose sufentanil for anesthesia and postoperative analgesia in neonatal cardiac surgery. New England Journal of Medicine 326:1–9.
6. Insel PA 1991 Analgesic-antipyretics and antiinflammatory agents; drugs employed in the treatment of rheumatoid arthritis and gout. In: Gilman AG, Rall TW, Nies AS, Taylor P (eds) Goodman and Gilman's The pharmacological basis of therapeutics, 8th edn. Pergamon Press, New York; pp. 617–657
7. Zaccara G, Muscas GC, Messori A 1990 Clinical features, pathogenesis and management of drug-induced seizures. Drug Safety 5:109–151
8. Spotoft H, Korshin JD, Sørensen MB, Skovsted P 1979 The cardiovascular effects of ketamine used for induction of anaesthesia in patients with valvular heart disease. Canadian Anaesthetists Society Journal 26:463–467

FURTHER READING

1. Tobias JD, Rasmussen GE 1994 Pain management and sedation in the pediatric intensive care unit. Pediatric Clinics of North America 41(6):1269–1292.
2. Park GR, Sladen RN (eds) 1995 Sedation and analgesia in the critically ill. Blackwell, Oxford

20

Accident and emergency care

Peter Barnett

INTRODUCTION

Children presenting to the emergency room (ER) with painful conditions require assessment of their pain, appropriate pain relief, and management of their underlying disease. Patient management must be based on a thorough assessment of not only the presenting disorder but also associated medical conditions and the patient's psychology, which will depend on developmental stage, family, and cultural factors. The distress of the pain and circumstances of the presenting condition may exaggerate fear of hospital procedures.

This chapter discusses pain management of common presentations to pediatric ERs. Topical, infiltration, and intravenous regional local anesthetic techniques are described. Nerve blocks, especially of the face and periphery, are useful for procedures in these areas and are described in Chapter 9. The use of other analgesics, such as acetaminophen (paracetamol), nitrous oxide and opioids, and sedation techniques as used in ERs are briefly described (see also Chs 3, 4, and 5). Appropriate psychological care, and good patient preparation and organization should supplement (and sometimes replace) pharmacological methods, and are briefly discussed (see also Ch. 13).

MANAGEMENT OF COMMON PAINFUL CONDITIONS AND PROCEDURES

Lacerations

Lacerations constitute 3% of all presentations to ERs. Most are superficial and commonly occur on the face, scalp, and extremities. Traditionally an uncooperative child was restrained, injected with a local anesthetic agent, and sutured, producing distress and fearful recollections. These problems can be avoided by selective use of alternative wound closure, other local anesthetic techniques, distraction techniques, and sedation or general anesthesia as required.

Local Anesthesia

Topical anesthesia is a common method either alone or preceding infiltration anesthesia. Careful technique (see below and Box 20.1) can minimize or eliminate the pain of producing local anesthesia. Nerve blocks and other regional anesthetic techniques (see below and also Ch. 9) may be useful in some patients.

Wound closure

Histoacryl tissue adhesive glue: Histoacryl tissue adhesive glue is an alternative to suture wound closure in suitable cases. The glue reacts with tissue fluid to form a polymer which takes approximately 30 seconds to set. It does not replace the need for deep sutures and is impossible to use in an environment which is constantly blood-stained as the glue will not adhere properly. Blood in the wound also increases the pain of the procedure. Compared with the use of sutures, tissue glue seems more acceptable to the patient and parents, has a similar cosmetic result, is faster, is relatively painless, and does not require sedation or later removal.[1]

To apply tissue glue, the wound is cleaned, the edges held together, and a small amount of glue (approximately 0.05 ml) placed along the line of the laceration. The wound edges are held together for 30 seconds. Skin closure strips should then be applied to prevent the child picking the glue off. The wound should be kept dry for 3–4 days and then washed. The scab will come off in 1–2 weeks.

Suturing: Appropriate local anesthesia, and occasionally sedation or general anesthesia, will be required for suturing. Using absorbable sutures on areas where the cosmetic advantages of polypropylene or nylon are not required (e.g. the scalp and hand) obviates the stress and potential pain of suture removal. Splinting any sutured wound that is under tension (e.g. across joints or on the hand) to remove the tension decreases pain and promotes healing.

Fractures

The management of common closed limb fractures has three phases, each with differing analgesia requirements. These stages are 'first-aid', including analgesia and splinting, definitive treatment with immobilization (and manipulation if required), and follow-up and prevention of complications. Appropriate use of rest, ice, compression, and elevation (RICE) will reduce swelling, which decreases pain and the risk of complications (see Ch. 13).

Initial management

The pain of fractures varies between patients. Usually the greater the degree of deformity, the more severe the pain. The first-aid management is splinting the limb to prevent movement of the fracture. This can be achieved by using a rolled-up newspaper or strapping a piece of wood to the affected limb. A simple sling (e.g. made from a shirt) may also immobilize the limb adequately. Immobilization provides analgesia and prevents further displacement of the fracture. In hospital a temporary plaster splint can be applied. It is best to do this after analgesia has been given.

In the ER, opioids are the mainstay of pharmacological treatment of acute pain due to a fracture. In the absence of interaction with other drugs (especially sedatives) or physical conditions (head injury, sleep apnea), respiratory depression or significant depression of conscious state are rare if dosage guidelines are followed. An opioid should be used unless the child appears comfortable and has no obvious deformity. Table 20.1 summarizes the doses of opioids commonly used in emergency departments.

Table 20.1   Opioids used in the emergency department

Drug	Dosage
Codeine	0.5–1.0 mg/kg oral
Meperidine	1–1.5 mg/kg i.m. or 0.5–1 mg/kg i.v.
Morphine	0.1–0.2 mg/kg i.m. or 0.05–0.1 mg/kg i.v.
Fentanyl	0.5–4 µg/kg i.v. or sublingually (not i.m.)

For patients with minor fractures, acetaminophen 20 mg/kg, with or without codeine 0.5–1 mg/kg, is usually satisfactory. This has an onset time of about half an hour. Intramuscular opioid is still preferred for more severe fractures, despite the moderate pain of injection, as it is more effective than codeine, can be given quickly, and is effective in about 15 minutes. Intravenous opioid analgesia has a faster onset and should be titrated using boluses of about one-fourth of the recommended intramuscular dose. Intravenous fentanyl has a rapid onset, with a greater potential for apnea than morphine owing to acutely high brain levels after a bolus. The relatively slower (several minutes) onset of intravenous morphine can result in excessive dosage if insufficient time is allowed between boluses. Formal splinting and radiography of the fracture should be delayed until effective analgesia has been achieved. Nausea and vomiting are the commonest adverse effects of opioids. Antiemetic use varies with age as vomiting is less frequent in small children. Generally, metoclopramide 0.1–0.2 mg/kg (maximum 15 mg) is used in children more than 8 years old. In patients with fractures and multitrauma (see below) analgesia should not be withheld but given intravenously and titrated to effect. Opioids will also have some anxiolytic effect and provide postoperative analgesia if manipulation is required.

Definitive treatment of fractures

For simple fractures a plaster cast or appropriate sling or strapping is all that is required. This will protect the limb from further damage or knocking and allow the fracture to heal. For displaced forearm fractures, manipulation and plaster are required. This can be performed under a local anesthetic block or general anesthesia. General anesthesia is usually required if (i) the child is less than 4–5 years old, (ii) venous access in the affected limb has been unsuccessful, (iii) the fracture is unstable after reduction, or (iv) open reduction is required. Generally plasters should be applied to immobilize the joint proximal and distal to the fracture.

Local anesthesia for fracture manipulation: For reduction of forearm fractures, intravenous regional block (IVRB) or 'Bier's block' is the usual anesthetic technique used for cooperative children aged about 5 years or more. It is uncommon to use the technique in the lower limb in children. The IVRB of the arm is described in detail below. Brachial plexus block, usually by the axillary route, has a place, but specialized training of the physician performing the block is required (see Ch. 9). The duration of plexus block is too long for most emergency outpatient procedures.

Hematoma block may be used if only one forearm bone is broken. With meticulous antisepsis and sterile technique, 5–10 ml of 1% lidocaine (maximum 5 mg/kg) is injected into the fracture. The major disadvantages are the pain of the injection and the risk of introducing bacteria into the fracture site.

Systemic analgesia when manipulating forearm fractures: Nitrous oxide inhalation (see Ch. 4) can be used for cooperative patients as young as 4 years.[2] Children need to be able to self-administer the gas. The smell of the circuit can be disguised using flavor mixtures which can be placed in the mask. Nitrous oxide analgesia is usually inadequate for manipulating a displaced fracture, but may assist casting or supplement inadequate local anesthesia.

An intravenous opioid and sedative can be used, but this is less than ideal as a large amount of opioid is usually required. This technique is not recommended unless managed in the same way as general anesthesia (see below) with appropriate personnel and facilities. After the manipulation, pain decreases and the opioid may produce delayed respiratory depression. This is exaggerated by the sedative drugs that must be given to achieve satisfactory operating conditions. Fentanyl or morphine are usually combined with midazolam. These agents may be used alone for anesthesia and analgesia, but are more useful (in low dose) as a supplement to local anesthesia.

Follow-up and prevention of complications

For 1–2 days after emergency treatment oral analgesia, such as acetaminophen 20 mg/kg alone or with codeine 0.5–1.0 mg/kg every 4–6 hours, is usually sufficient. The patient should be instructed to contact the ER if pain is severe or not sufficiently relieved by these oral analgesics.

Older children with forearm fractures should be advised to keep the affected limb elevated above the heart (e.g. on the patient's head while walking around or on several pillows when sitting down) for the first 24 hours. A sling should *not* be worn during this time as this makes the limb dependent. Written instructions on plaster care should be given to parents. These should include warning signs of vascular compromise of the limb. If these signs occur (e.g. blue, cold, numb, painful, or swollen digits) then the limb should be elevated for half an hour. If no relief occurs, the plaster usually needs to be split. Medical review the day after plaster application is recommended to check if the plaster is too tight.

Intravenous cannulation

Lidocaine (lignocaine) and prilocaine cream (Emla) or 4% tetracaine (amethocaine) gel can provide suitable anesthesia of the skin when properly used (placed over the injection site under an occlusive dressing about 60 minutes prior to the procedure).[3] The idea of venipuncture is so frightening for some, especially younger children, that various nonpharmacological techniques may be crucial for minimizing distress (see below and Ch. 13).

Calico dolls have been used to prepare children for painful procedures, such as intravenous cannulation. These dolls are plain dolls that have no features. The nurse or person preparing the child for the procedure first allows the child to 'make' their own doll by coloring it. Once the child 'owns' the doll, then the nurse assistant will explain the planned procedure to the child using the doll as the patient. The child may participate in the procedure, for example by putting a pretend needle into the doll or suturing the doll, although this is usually done by the nurse. This preparation helps explain to the child what is about to happen. Ideally, the actual procedure should be nearly painless, as pain will cause the child to lose confidence in the staff. Meticulous use of local anesthesia as described above is often the best means of achieving this. Calico dolls can also be used to distract children during examination, keep them occupied during their stay in the ER, and to make their memory of their hospital experience more positive.

Lumbar puncture

Topical local anesthesia with lidocaine and prilocaine cream or 4% tetracaine gel followed by local anesthetic (e.g. 1% lidocaine) infiltration should prevent pain due to lumbar puncture. Holding the child in the correct position decreases the chance of the needle hitting bone, which is painful. In infants under 6 months old a sharp 23 gauge hypodermic needle without stylet can be used without infiltration anesthetic with minimal pain, but there is a small risk of introducing a piece of skin into the spinal canal causing infection or an inclusion dermoid.

Nasal foreign body removal

Topical phenylephrine (0.5%) and lidocaine (5%) spray on the nasal mucosa will produce both anesthesia and vasoconstriction, allowing better access to the foreign body. Care must be taken to keep the doses of these agents within the maximum allowed (7 mg/kg lidocaine with phenylephrine, 2 mg/kg cocaine), especially in small children.

Suprapubic aspirate

Analgesia is rarely used for suprapubic aspiration procedures as the opportunity to perform the test outweighs the advantage of waiting for topical anesthetic cream to work. Small children void frequently, so suprapubic aspiration should be performed approximately 20–30 minutes after the last void. Use a 23 gauge needle attached to a 2 ml or 5 ml syringe.

Earache

Earache is a common presentation to pediatric ERs. It can be extremely distressing to the child and is usually due to otitis media. Perforation of the eardrum (spontaneous or surgical) relieves the pain of otitis media which is caused by the pressure of the middle ear fluid collection. Both topical and systemic analgesics can be used for acute earache.

Topical treatment can be given using 1% lidocaine solution or a thick solution of benzocaine and phenazone (Auralgin otic) applied directly into the ear canal. The patient should then lie on their side (affected side up) for approximately 10 minutes to allow the solution to reach the eardrum; moving the tragus backwards and forwards may help to achieve this. The analgesia lasts 1–2 hours and the application can be repeated every 2 hours.[4] Acetaminophen in adequate dosage is usually an effective analgesic for earache. The dose should be 20 mg/kg with a maximum of 100 mg/kg per day. A dose of 30 mg/kg is useful as a loading dose or at bedtime to give longer pain relief. After this larger dose, no more acetaminophen should be given for at least 6 hours to avoid high peak plasma levels. The addition of codeine (0.5–1.0 mg/kg) may be helpful if acetaminophen alone is inadequate. Suitable proprietary pediatric acetaminophen and codeine mixtures are available in many countries. Mixtures with promethazine may also have a role, especially for nocturnal sedation in the patient with earache.

Nonpharmacological relief of earache may also be produced by warm compresses held over the ear. Using a hair-dryer on a low setting to blow warm air into the ear canal may also be helpful.

Eye injuries

Corneal abrasions and burns can be extremely painful. The use of topical anesthesia (e.g. tetracaine 0.5% eye-drops) will initially relieve pain to allow a thorough assessment. It is important not to continue to use tetracaine as this is toxic to the corneal epithelium with repeated use, and the corneal anesthesia may lead to inadvertent abrasion or undiagnosed foreign bodies in the eye causing further corneal damage. After assessment of the eye, antibiotic ointment should be placed on the cornea and a double eye-patch placed to avoid blinking which produces more pain. Corneal abrasion may produce reflex spasm of the iris, causing pain which may be relieved by topical atropine.

Multiple trauma

Patients who present with multiple trauma are usually in pain. Adequate analgesia is part of their secondary survey and management. The primary assessment must ensure that the patient's airway, breathing, and circulation are adequate prior to analgesia. Monitoring should be continuous to detect possible change in the underlying pathological condition, adequacy of resuscitation, and complications of the analgesia such as hypoventilation. Intravenous opioid agonists such as morphine or fentanyl should be titrated using small boluses in hypovolemic patients (e.g. 0.02–0.05 mg/kg morphine), because the reduced blood volume and increased proportion of cardiac output going to the brain makes apnea more likely. Equipment for artificial ventilation and naloxone should be available should apnea or marked respiratory depression occur. An antiemetic may be required in older children.

Administration of opioids intramuscularly, subcutaneously, or via the gastrointestinal tract is relatively contraindicated in children who are hypovolemic. Hypovolemia causes a marked decrease in blood flow to muscle, skin, and the gastrointestinal tract, which markedly reduces the rate of opioid uptake by these routes. The lack of effect that this produces may encourage the inappropriate administration of repeat doses which will act as a large depot of opioid. When the patient is resuscitated, improved blood flow to these organs may produce rapid uptake of this depot producing delayed respiratory depression. Local anesthesia may be useful, producing profound analgesia without sedation, respiratory depression, or nausea and vomiting. A good example is the use of femoral nerve blockade (see Ch. 9) for proximal femur fractures.

LOCAL AND REGIONAL ANESTHESIA

Local and regional anesthetic techniques are also discussed in Chapter 9.

Lidocaine

Lidocaine 0.5–2% injectable has a rapid onset, short duration, and an excellent safety and efficacy record. Its disadvantages are that it is a painful injection and it may distort the area to be sutured. There are simple measures to decrease the pain involved in injecting lidocaine (Box 20.1). Epinephrine (adrenaline) 1:100 000 (10 μg/ml) to 1:200 000 (5 μg/ml) added to lidocaine prolongs anesthesia and reduces bleeding. Epinephrine is contraindicated around end arteries, such as in digits and the penis. The prepackaged solutions are more acidic (and painful) than solutions to which the operator adds the epinephrine. The addition of 1 ml of sodium bicarbonate 8.4% to 9 ml of lidocaine 1% (even without epinephrine) produces a less acidic solution, with faster onset (owing to a greater percentage of unionized drug being available), which is less painful to inject.[5] This solution is stable for 24 hours only. The maximum dose of lidocaine for neural blockade is 5 mg/kg or 8 mg/kg with epinephrine. Inadvertent intravascular injection should be carefully avoided, as much smaller amounts than the recommended maximum doses of lidocaine may cause seizures and cardiac arrest if given intravascularly. Tinnitus, perioral paresthesia and generalized muscle twitching may be a prodrome to more serious local anesthetic toxicity (see below).

Box 20.1 Measures that decrease the pain of infiltration anesthesia

Use topical anesthesia first
Use a fine needle (27 to 32 gauge)
Inject slowly
Place the needle into the wound through the lacerated surface, not through intact
  skin
Pass the needle via the anesthetized area into the unanesthetized area
Lidocaine 1% is effective and less painful than the 2% solution
Buffer lidocaine with sodium bicarbonate (see text)

Topical anesthesia

Several topical anesthesia solutions and gels have been used since the 1980s. The first was a mixture of tetracaine 2%, adrenaline (epinephrine) 1:2000, and cocaine 11.8% (TAC). Many controlled trials have shown an efficacy of 90–95% on facial and scalp wounds but only approximately 50% on limb wounds.[6] This is due to poorer skin blood supply in limbs. Topical TAC can be applied in a solution or gel (solution mixed with methylcellulose). The mixture should never be used on mucous membranes, lips, the inner aspect of the nose, or the eyelid, as there have been several reports of death due to its rapid absorption across mucous membranes. The use of TAC is contraindicated in end artery areas (e.g. ear, fingers, tip of nose, penis) as its profound vasoconstrictor effects may produce ischemia.

The maximum dose of TAC (topical only) is 1 ml per 10 kg body weight. It should be applied to cotton wool which is then moulded to the shape of the wound and placed inside the wound as much as possible. This is held in place with adhesive tape (or often by a parent) for at least 10–15 minutes. An area of blanching approximately 1 cm wide will appear around the wound. Adequacy of anesthesia should then be tested by washing the wound and squeezing the wound together. If no pain is elicited with these maneuvres then suturing will usually be painless. The sensation of pulling and light touch are preserved and this should be explained to the child and parent. The anesthesia lasts for about 1 hour.

Similar results have been achieved with newer, less toxic topical preparations. The first of these was 'half TAC' which contained only 4% cocaine. This still had the problems of the high cost of the medication (particularly cocaine) and the need for secure storage. A combination of 1:2000 adrenaline (epinephrine) and 11.8% cocaine (AC) has been used with success. However, lignocaine 4%, adrenaline (epinephrine) 1:1000, and tetracaine 0.5% (LAT) has been shown to be as effective as TAC but at a tenth of the cost, and without the administrative problems of cocaine.[7]

Tetracaine 4% gel without epinephrine or cocaine and a eutectic mixture of 5% lidocaine and prilocaine (Emla cream, Astra) were designed for use on unbroken skin, but in one study[8] they have successfully (and safely) been used on open wounds (despite the Emla product information warning against this because of the risk of increased systemic absorption). The advantage of these products is better anesthesia of extremity wounds, but their slow onset of action (approximately 45–60 minutes) is a disadvantage. It is important to remove all the cream from the wound by irrigation prior to suturing to minimize the risk of wound infection.

Nerve blocks

Nerve blocks can be used for analgesia but are more commonly used as anesthesia for laceration repair or manipulation of fractures. Nerve blocks tend to be underused in pediatrics, but most are simple to perform and provide excellent analgesia and anesthesia. For example, fractures of the metacarpal of the fifth (little) finger can be reduced under ulnar nerve block. A number of nerve blocks are described in Chapter 9. Those involving the distal limbs and face are particularly useful in the ER.

Lidocaine 1% has a rapid onset, short duration, and is adequate for most blocks in ERs. Lidocaine 2% can speed the onset and produce a denser block, especially when larger nerves are being anesthetized. Bupivacaine 0.25% and 0.5% solutions are equivalent, but have a slower onset and longer duration. The long duration prolongs analgesia but raises concern about discharging patients with anesthetized areas that may be inadvertently traumatized. The use of topical local anesthesia prior to injection, fine needles (or even anesthetizing the skin and subcutaneous tissues if a short beveled needle, see Ch. 9, is used for the block), and slow injection can minimize the pain of the block. Care should be taken not to inject against resistance, to avoid nerve injury. Massage of the area after injection will often improve the spread of the local anesthetic solution.

Intravenous regional block (Bier's block)

Intravenous regional block (IVRB) or Bier's block is a straightforward procedure which if performed correctly has excellent results.[9,10] It involves intravenous injection of local anesthetic drug into the affected arm under arterial tourniquet. *The tourniquet must be maintained for a minimum of 20 minutes after the local anesthetic injection*, even if the procedure is brief. This allows time for the local anesthetic solution to penetrate the tissues, slowing washout and preventing potentially toxic blood levels when the tourniquet is released. The *tourniquet cuff pressure must be continuously monitored until it is time to release it*. The block should only be performed by suitably accredited medical staff with appropriate equipment and training to deal with complications. Bupivacaine is absolutely contraindicated for this block owing to the greater risk of cardiac arrest should early cuff failure produce acute systemic toxicity. Prilocaine or lidocaine are the drugs of choice.

When a child with an injury (particularly a forearm fracture) suitable for repair under IVRB first presents to the ER, appropriate analgesia is given and a topical anesthetic cream is applied to the back of each hand. After assessment, obtaining informed consent and allowing enough time for the topical anesthesia to take effect, IVRB can commence. Intravenous access is obtained via a cannula on the unaffected arm and by cannula or butterfly needle on the affected arm. An appropriately sized inflatable cuff is then put around the affected limb, which is held above the heart to allow drainage of venous blood from the arm. The cuff is then inflated to approximately 200 mgHg (at least 60 mmHg above systolic pressure). It is crucial that the cuff pressure is monitored and maintained, and that the cuff cannot loosen or disconnect. The tubing between the manometer and the cuff must not be clamped. Lidocaine or prilocaine 3 mg/kg (0.6 ml/kg of 0.5% solution) is injected intravenously distal to the arterial tourniquet. The arm will become blotchy (cutis marmorata, due to patchy redistribution of blood from deep to superficial veins) and the patient will usually experience a sensation of warmth in the limb. Onset of anesthesia takes about 5–10 minutes. With a successful block, a fracture can be manipulated without pain. When reducing a fracture under IVRB, the plaster is applied and a check X-ray taken before the cuff is deflated in case remanipulation is required. The cuff should *not* be let down until at least 20 minutes after the local anesthetic solution has been injected.

Tourniquet pain is the most common minor side-effect. Most children will tolerate the cuff for 20–25 minutes, which is sufficient time for most procedures. Although it increases the complexity of the procedure and the pneumatic connections – and thus the risk of early cuff failure – some operators use a double cuff technique to prevent tourniquet pain, especially if a more prolonged procedure is planned. Two cuffs are placed on the limb. The proximal cuff is inflated and local anesthetic solution injected as for the single cuff technique. After 5 minutes the distal cuff is inflated over what is now an anesthetized part of the arm. After checking that the distal cuff is functioning correctly, the proximal cuff may be deflated. The distal cuff acts as the tourniquet till the end of the procedure, and is deflated after the usual minimum 20 minutes.

Complications of local anesthesia

Local anesthetic toxicity, usually due to early cuff failure in IVRB or accidental intravascular injection during nerve blocks, may cause seizures sometimes preceded by tinnitus, muscle twitching, or perioral paresthesia. Apnea, dysrhythmia, and cardiac arrest can occur. Management of a seizure involves maintenance of the airway, assisted ventilation with oxygen, and monitoring of oxygenation and the circulation. The seizures are usually brief. If prolonged, a benzodiazepine or thiopentone may be required but may cause apnea. Although rare, local anesthetic toxicity from cuff failure is so potentially serious that trained medical staff and facilities to deal with this event must always be available when an IVRB is performed.

SEDATION AND GENERAL ANESTHESIA

Sedation is commonly used to facilitate procedures performed in the ER. It will often be supplemented by local anesthesia. Careful monitoring and drug titration are required to avoid deeper levels of sedation than desired, and staff and facilities must be able to cope with an unconscious patient (see below). Some centres will have the resources to perform general anesthesia within the ER, usually in a purpose-built operating room. Management of these patients should be under the supervision of a trained anesthesiologist. Stomach emptying is impaired by trauma, and fasting is often inadequate or unreliable. Most emergency patients should be treated as if they have a full stomach.

Sedation

Conscious sedation is the level of sedation most frequently used in the ER. Conscious sedation is present when there is minimal depression of the level of consciousness, protective reflexes are intact (e.g. cough, gag), and the patient has appropriate responses to command or mildly painful stimuli. Monitoring should be performed by the physician doing the procedure with the help of an adequately trained nurse. If deep sedation occurs, (sleep or unconsciousness), then the operating physician should attend to the patient monitoring and general care until another physician is available or the patient returns to a conscious sedated state. Monitoring and resuscitation equipment required for conscious sedation are listed in Boxes 20.2 and 20.3.

Box 20.2 Monitoring required for conscious sedation

Continuous:
  Conscious state
  Respiration
  Heart rate
  HbO_2 saturation

Intermittent:
  Respiratory rate
  Blood pressure
  Patient restraint (if used)
  Documentation of drugs given

> **Box 20.3**   Equipment required for conscious sedation
>
> Oxygen and delivery systems
> Suction
> Equipment for assisted ventilation
> Oximeter
> Automatic blood pressure cuff
> Full equipment for cardiopulmonary resuscitation

Deep sedation may occur inadvertently during conscious sedation or as one method of anesthesia. Deep sedation involves loss of communication with the patient and is associated with loss of protective reflexes. Deep sedation should be managed and assessed as if the patient were under general anesthesia. Whenever conscious sedation is undertaken, because of the risk of deep sedation occurring, experienced staff who have advanced life support skills should be immediately available and equipment for advanced cardiopulmonary resuscitation should be checked and on hand.

General anesthesia

General anesthesia involves a wide range of possible techniques which may be conducted by an appropriately trained anesthesiologist, with an anesthetist assistant and suitable facilities for monitoring and resuscitation. The person performing the procedure for which the child requires anesthesia must not be the anesthesiologist. There must be good perioperative communication between the operator and the anesthesiologist so that the planning of appropriate techniques, and timing of the surgery and anesthesia are based on the full clinical assessment of all the clinicians involved.

CONCLUSION

The management of pain and distress in the ER depends on the pathological condition involved, the age and understanding of the child, and the expertise of the physician looking after the patient. Any patient in pain should be treated promptly and the treatment should include appropriate pain management.

REFERENCES

1. Jarman F, McGill K, Aickin R, Goodge J, Silk G, Barnett P 1995 Randomised trial of tissue adhesive glue vs suturing for the repair of pediatric lacerations Archives of Pediatric and Adolescent Medicine 149:77
2. Wattenmaker I, Kasser JR, McGravey A 1990 Self-administered nitrous oxide for fracture reduction in children in an emergency room setting. Journal of Orthopedic Trauma 4(1):35–38
3. Hopkins CS, Buckley CJ, Bush GH 1988 Pain free injection in infants. Use of a lignocaine-prilocaine cream to prevent pain at intravenous induction of general anesthesia in 1–5 year old children. Anaesthesia 43(3):198–201

4. Hoberman A, Paradise JL, Reynolds E, Urkin J 1995 Efficacy of Auralgan for ear pain in children with acute otitis media. Pediatric Research 37(4):137A
5. Steinbrook RA, Hughes N, Fanciullo G, Manzi D, Ferrante FM 1993 Effects of alkalinization of lidocaine on the pain of skin infiltration and intravenous catheterization. Journal of Clinical Anesthesia 5(6):456–458
6. Heganbarth MA, Altieri MF, Hawk WH, Greene A, Ochsenschlager DW, O'Donnell R 1990 Comparison of topical tetracaine, adrenaline, and cocaine anesthesia with lidocaine infiltration for the repair of lacerations in children. Annals of Emergency Medicine 19(1):63–67
7. Schilling CG, Bank DE, Borchart BA, Klatzko MD, Uden DL 1995 Tetracaine, epinephrine (adrenalin), and cocaine (TAC) versus lidocaine, epinephrine and tetracaine for anesthesia of lacerations in children. Annals of Emergency Medicine 25(2):203–208
8. Zempsky WT, Karasic RB 1995 Superiority of EMLA compared with TAC for topical anesthesia of extremity wounds in children. Archives of Pediatric and Adolescent Medicine 149:59
9. Colizza WA, Said E 1993 Intravenous regional anesthesia in the treatment of forearm and wrist fractures and dislocations in children. Canadian Journal of Surgery 36(3):225–228
10. Lowen R, Taylor J 1994 Bier's block – the experience of Australian emergency departments. Medical Journal of Australia 160:108–111

21 Pain in pediatric rheumatologic disorders

Roger Allen

INTRODUCTION

A wide variety of painful conditions in childhood, both inflammatory and noninflammatory, affect joints. The principles of pain management are common to all the arthritides, but details of management and prognosis will vary with the precise diagnosis (see below). The four principles listed here are discussed below.

- Use of basic analgesic strategies
- Control of the inflammatory process
- Maintaining joint function
- Use of age-appropriate behavioral intervention

A number of common noninflammatory pediatric rheumatological conditions are discussed at the end of this chapter.

CLASSIFICATION OF IDIOPATHIC ARTHRITIDES

Juvenile chronic arthritis (JCA), is the most common form of persistent arthritis in childhood, affecting approximately 1 in 1500 children less than 16 years of age. It is not a homogeneous disease and the criteria for subclassification remain the topic of current international discussion.[1] One recent classification describes the following seven clinical entities based on onset, associated features, number of joints affected, and whether the joints were affected in the first 6 months of the disease.

1. *Systemic onset*: arthritis with typical evanescent rash and quotidian fever
2. *Polyarthritis – rheumatoid factor negative*: affects more than four joints in first 6 months
3. *Polyarthritis – rheumatoid factor positive*: affects more than four joints in first 6 months
4. *Oligoarthritis* – affects one to four joints during first 6 months of disease
5. *Extended oligoarthritis* – only progresses to more than four joints after 6 months
6. *Enthesitis-related* – inflammation at ligamentous insertions in addition to arthritis
7. *Psoriatic arthritis*

The enthesitis-related arthropathy typically has spondyloarthropathy-related features and may progress to ankylosing spondylitis. Excluded from the classification above are a variety of other chronic inflammatory arthritides such as those which are features of more specific disorders, e.g. systemic lupus erythematosus and related connective tissue diseases, and arthritis associated with other chronic disorders, e.g. inflammatory bowel disease and cystic fibrosis.

PAIN MANAGEMENT

The management of pain is one of the most challenging aspects of chronic forms of juvenile arthritis.[2,3] Previously there was a perception that inflammatory arthritis did not produce pain to the same extent in children, particularly of preschool age, as in adolescents or adults.[4] Pain expression may be age-related. For example, a toddler may not complain of pain due to an inflamed knee but may withdraw from normal walking, preferring to be carried, or may keep the affected site flexed to reduce the intraarticular pressure. It is important to recognize the protective mechanisms that a child may use to overcome pain, adopting particular joint positions and modifying function. To ignore these may lead to inappropriate and possibly irreversible joint changes as well as to functional disability.[5] It has been postulated that the 'meaning' children attribute to a painful sensation from involved joints influences the degree of pain perceived. As older children and adolescents associate the internal sensations with an actual understanding of a pathological process they are more likely to consider the sensation 'painful'.[6] Disease duration and effective adaptation may also relate to pain behavior. While children with JCA describe more pain sensations as they reach adolescence, this is particularly so in children who were relatively older at the onset of their disease.[7] This may reflect better understanding of pathology, but may involve the psychologic issues of 'loss' at such a formative time in a child's emotional development.

Nociceptive responses in articular and surrounding tissues are transmitted by Aδ (type III) and C (type IV) fibers (see Ch. 2). These will be stimulated by physical factors (exceeding the normal joint range, pressure, or heat) or chemical factors (inflammatory mediators such as bradykinins, histamine, and cytokines). The degree of inflammation indicated by synovial fluid neutrophil count and erythrocyte sedimentation rate has been reported as lower in children with less pain behavior, implying a link between inflammation and pain.[8] Correlation of pain levels with physiological parameters such as joint temperature, assessed by thermography, has been inconsistent.[9] Prostaglandin synthesis induced by inflammation (see Ch. 2) is inhibited by nonsteroidal antiinflammatory drugs (NSAIDs). Prostaglandins contribute to hyperalgesia indirectly by sensitizing nociceptive nerve endings to respond to previously nonpainful stimuli and by synergism with the other inflammatory mediators in their chemical nociceptive capacity.[10]

Inflammation may alter firing thresholds for the various nociceptive receptors, and JCA patients have lower pain thresholds to pressure algometers applied to joints or paravertebral structures compared with controls.[11] Patients with JCA in remission demonstrate lower pain thresholds than controls, suggesting that 'central sensitization' occurs. It is postulated that repetitive nociceptive input during the period of active inflammation alters the responsiveness of second-order neurons so that these neurons transmitting nociceptive stimuli now respond to nonnociceptive stimuli generated by type II ($A\beta$) afferents. Minimizing pain from the onset of JCA may limit this effect, improving the patient's future pain experience.

Basic analgesic strategies

Unfortunately, increased episodes of pain may occur even with well-controlled arthritis. Usually simple analgesia such as acetaminophen (paracetamol) in standard doses will be sufficient. For intermittent analgesia, salicylates still have a role at lower dosage levels (10–15 mg/kg per dose). Concerns over Reye syndrome, hepatic toxicity, and the inconvenience of the short duration of action of salicylates, make other NSAIDs more popular as standard antiinflammatory therapy. In more resistant pain the use of acetaminophen–codeine combination preparations may be useful. Long-term combined use of acetaminophen and NSAIDs has been associated with acute renal tubular necrosis owing to metabolism to phenacetin, and should be avoided.[12]

Low-dose NSAID preparations are available as nonprescription analgesics (e.g. ibuprofen 200 mg per dose). The role of such preparations for patients already taking antiinflammatory doses of an NSAID has not been evaluated although clinical experience suggests they may be of assistance, particularly as combining NSAIDs of different classes is sometimes useful. Topical NSAID preparations have been widely used in sports medicine and have been found useful for localized pain in some adolescent JCA patients.

Physical therapies (see below and Ch. 13) include a wide range of methods which may be selected according to the type and site of the pain. For example, warm or hot packs can be applied to individual joints, and warm baths may be useful. Compressive insoles can relieve metatarsal or calcaneal pain, particularly in those with enthesitic pain. Periods of physical rest may be valuable but need to be closely monitored. Joint symptoms such as pain, and even signs of swelling, may improve with bed rest; however, this may be at the expense of other aspects of joint function such as position and muscle strength. Rest therefore needs to be a carefully designed part of a child's program and coupled with active physical therapy.

Control of the inflammatory process

Control of inflammation is the primary focus of both disease and pain management. Antiinflammatory drugs can be considered in four groups (Table 21.1): nonsteroidal antiinflammatory drugs, slow-acting antirheumatic drugs (SAARDs), immunosuppressants, and corticosteroids, both oral and intraarticular. The mechanism by which these therapies modify pain is probably by suppression of inflammatory mediators. The response time is variable between agents, the route of delivery, and

Table 21.1   Drug dosages for juvenile chronic arthritis

Drug	Daily dose	Dosage schedule
Nonsteroidal antiinflammatory drugs		
Aspirin	60–100 mg/kg	3–4 times daily
Naproxen	15 mg/kg	Twice daily
Diclofenac	2.5 mg/kg	Twice daily
Ibuprofen	40 mg/kg	3 times daily
Indomethacin	2.5 mg/kg	3 times daily
Piroxicam	0.5 mg/kg	Once daily
Slow-acting Antirheumatic drugs		
Hydroxychloroquine	6 mg/kg	Once daily
Sulfasalazine	40 mg/kg	Twice daily
Penicillamine	10 mg/kg	Twice daily
Auranofin	0.15 mg/kg	Twice daily
Gold	1 mg/kg	Weekly
Immunosuppressants		
Methotrexate	10 mg/m^2	Weekly
Azathioprine	2 mg/kg	Twice daily
Corticosteroids		
Prednisolone	Aim for < 0.5 mg/kg	Alternate days
Triamcinolone hexacetonide (or acetonide)		Dose related to joint size

the disease onset subtype. For example, intraarticular corticosteroids produce a rapid antiinflammatory response of variable duration.[13] Intraarticular therapy is rarely indicated for pain alone, particularly in young children for whom the procedure may require general anesthesia.

The time taken for an adequate antiinflammatory response to NSAIDs can vary between individuals and may depend on some longer-acting properties of these agents.[14] Overall there is little difference between the various NSAIDs in their antiinflammatory efficacy in JCA.[15] An NSAID may produce rapid analgesia despite the signs of inflammation taking weeks to resolve. Therefore if pain has been adequately controlled, it is appropriate to continue an NSAID for 6–8 weeks before it is decided that its antiinflammatory effect is inadequate.

The role of second-line agents, particularly sulfasalazine or methotrexate, is for unresponsive JCA or in the severe polyarticular onset forms, in which case there is usually little value in awaiting the NSAID response before introducing these agents. Their role is directed solely at inflammatory control, and although this relates to pain, they have no direct role in pain control.

All drugs used in JCA management have toxicities that need to be considered and usage weighed up against the severity and subtype of disease. Monitoring for the complications of these drugs is crucial for their safe use. Gastric intolerance is particularly common with NSAIDs. Tests for hepatic, renal, and hematologic complications of the SAARDs and NSAIDs should be performed regularly. Growth and the onset of osteoporosis should be monitored in patients on corticosteroids.

Maintenance of joint position and function

The development of flexion contractures is common in juvenile arthritis if measures directed at maintaining appropriate joint alignment are not taken. Children with joint effusions adopt a position of flexion of that joint. This minimizes the intraarticular pressure and relieves pain, but fixed flexion deformities may result. Physiotherapists and occupational therapists must recognize behavior that relieves pain but worsens joint function,[16] and design their treatment programs to maximize function while minimizing pain. Splinting, stretching and strengthening exercises, assessment of aids and orthotics, and shoe raises for leg length discrepancy may all be used.

Behavioral and psychological interventions in pain management

It is important to acknowledge the age variation of children with JCA and that the concept of 'pain' may have little meaning to a young child in the preabstract stage of cognitive development. This fact has contributed to the concept that pain is not as significant a problem in the young JCA patient as it is in adolescents or adults. A number of pain scoring techniques have been used, including visual analog scales and faces[17] (see Ch. 10), but the most developed assessment for the JCA population is the Varni–Thompson pediatric pain questionnaire (PPQ).[18] The PPQ includes a 10 cm visual analog scale, a body outline on which the child localizes sites of pain using self-selected color grading of severity, and a selection of pain descriptors to assess sensory, affective, and evaluative qualities of pain perception. Parents also complete a similar assessment which includes aspects of family pain history and other socioenvironmental features that may influence both the child's and the parent's perception of the child's pain level and functional status. Using this tool, 72% of the variance of pain in children's reporting of worst pain severity was due to the child's psychological adjustment, family psychosocial environment, and disease parameters.[19]

Given the effect of psychological adjustment and family psychosocial environment on pain in children with JCA, it is not surprising that cognitive behavior therapy has been successful in these patients. Originally developed for patients with hemophiliac arthropathy, the program consists of progressive muscle relaxation, meditative breathing exercises, and age-appropriate guided imagery (see Ch. 13). Guided imagery can produce not only distraction but also thought diversion to pleasant experiences and to images representing a metaphor for the sensory pain experience. By imagination the child aims to alter the metaphor and therefore the pain perception. For example, the heat and pain of a joint could be pictured as a blowtorch that can be extinguished. Follow-up over 6–12 months found consistent decreases in pain and improved adaptive functioning.[20]

NONINFLAMMATORY RHEUMATOLOGIC DISORDERS

A variety of noninflammatory musculoskeletal disorders usually present with pain,[21] including benign nocturnal limb pain (growing pains), benign hypermobility-associated pain, patellofemoral dysfunction (anterior knee pain syndromes), and juvenile fibrositis (fibromyalgia).

Nocturnal limb pains

Nocturnal limb pains are common in children aged 4–8 years, and usually affect the knee, shin, and calf. No inflammatory features are present, although in the author's experience hypermobility is common in younger children whereas hamstring muscle tightness is often present in older cases. Other causes of bone pain, particularly acute leukemia, warrant consideration, but the lack of other signs and relief with simple massage and acetaminophen indicate the benign nature of the condition. The episodes are self-limited, but the parents and child need strong reassurance as the pains may persist for months to years.

Benign hypermobility

Benign hypermobility is a common finding in children in the preteenage group presenting with arthralgia typically occurring in the afternoon or after activity. Inflammatory features are absent, although bland knee effusions may be present notably after prolonged physical activities.[22] In the adolescent group hypermobility may also be found in conjunction with low back pain and patellofemoral abnormalities. Treatment is usually symptomatic but attention to muscle-strengthening exercises and simple orthoses for plantar arch support may assist.

Anterior patellofemoral pain

Anterior patellofemoral pain is common, particularly in adolescents. With the increased use of arthroscopy it has become apparent that the term chondromalacia patellae is overused in these situations, as macroscopically the cartilage looks normal. The nature of the pain and its management are the same as in chondromalacia, consisting of quadriceps strengthening, concentrating on the medial muscles, avoiding aggravating activities and medial strapping of the patella to assist correct alignment.[23] A useful guide to the correct diagnosis is the initiation of the pain with patella compression exacerbated further by resisted quadriceps contraction (positive apprehension sign).

Fibromyalgia– fibrositis syndrome

Fibromyalgia–fibrositis syndrome occurs particularly in teenage girls. Owing to a subjective sense of joint 'swelling', morning stiffness, and a general sense of ill-health, such patients may be labeled as having an 'inflammatory arthritis' and inappropriately treated. Importantly, patients have no objective synovitis but demonstrate tender areas within specific muscle bellies, so-called 'trigger points'. Other symptoms include fatigue, chronic anxiety, nonrestorative sleep, and often features of other pain syndromes such as chronic headache and irritable bowel syndrome.[24] Treatment requires a combination of explanation and reassurance, graded physiotherapy, antiinflammatory medication for analgesia and antidepressant therapy for improved sleep, and psychologic evaluation.[21] Behavioral cognitive approaches to pain management may assist some of these patients.

REFERENCES

1. Fink CW 1995 Proposal for the development of classification criteria for idiopathic arthritides of childhood. Journal of Rheumatology 22:1566–1569

2. Lovell DJ, Walco GA 1989 Pain associated with juvenile rheumatoid arthritis. Pediatric Clinics of North America 36:1015–1027
3. Varni JW 1992 Evaluation and management of pain in children with juvenile rheumatoid arthritis. Journal of Rheumatology 19(suppl. 33):32–35
4. Laaksonen AL, Laine V 1961 A comparative study of joint pain in adult and juvenile rheumatoid arthritis. Annals of Rheumatic Disease 20:386–387
5. Truckenbrodt H 1990 Pain in juvenile chronic arthritis: consequences for the musculoskeletal system. Clinical Experimental Rheumatology 11(suppl. 9):S59–S63
6. Beales JG, Holt PJ, Keen JH, Mellor VP 1983 Children with juvenile chronic arthritis: their beliefs about their illness and therapy. Annals of Rheumatic Disease 42:481–486
7. Hagglund KJ, Schopp LM, Alberts KR, Cassidy JT, Frank RG 1995 Predicting pain among children with juvenile rheumatoid arthritis. Arthritis Care Research 8:36–42
8. Sherry DD, Bohnsack J, Salmonson K, Wallace CA, Mellins E 1990 Painless juvenile rheumatoid arthritis. Journal of Pediatrics 116:921–923
9. Ilowite NT, Walco GA, Pochaczevsky R 1992 Assessment of pain in patients with juvenile rheumatoid arthritis: relation between pain intensity and degree of joint inflammation. Annals of Rheumatic Disease 51:343–346
10. Maunuksela E-L 1993 Nonsteroidal anti-inflammatory drugs in pediatric pain management. In: Schechter NL, Berde CB, Yaster M (eds) Pain in infants, children, and adolescents. Willams & Wilkins, Baltimore, p 135
11. Hogeweg JA, Kuis W, Huygen ACJ et al 1995 The pain threshold in juvenile chronic arthritis. British Journal of Rheumatology 34:61–67
12. Allen RC, Petty RE, Lirenman DS, Malleson PN, Laxer RM 1986 Renal papillary necrosis in children with chronic arthritis. American Journal of Diseases of Children 140:20–22
13. Allen RC, Gross KR, Beauchamp R, Malleson PN, Laxer RM, Petty RE 1986 Intra-articular use of triamcinolone hexacetonide in juvenile arthritis. Arthritis and Rheumatism 29:997–1001
14. Lovell DJ, Giannini EH, Brewer EJ 1984 Time course of response to nonsteroidal antiinflammatory drugs in juvenile rheumatoid arthritis. Arthritis and Rheumatism 27:1433-1437
15. Leak AM, Richter MR, Clemens LE et al 1988 A cross-over study of naproxen, diclofenac and tolmetin in seronegative juvenile chronic arthritis. Clinical Experimental and Rheumatology 6:157–160
16. Jaworski TM 1993 Juvenile rheumatoid arthritis: pain-related and psychosocial aspects and their relevance for assessment and treatment. Arthritis Care Research 6:187–196
17. Bieiri D, Reeve RA, Champion GD, Addicoat L, Ziegler JB 1990 The faces pain scale for the self-assessment of the severity of pain experienced by children. Pain 41:139–150
18. Varni JW, Thompson KL 1985 The Varni/Thompson pediatric pain questionnaire.
19. Varni JW, Thompson KL, Hanson V 1987 The Varni/Thompson pediatric pain questionnaire. I: Chronic musculoskeletal pain in juvenile rheumatoid arthritis. Pain 28:27–38
20. Walco GA, Varni JW, Ilowite NT 1992 Cognitive-behavioral pain management in children with juvenile rheumatoid arthritis. Pediatrics 89:1075–1079
21. Allen RC 1993 Differential diagnosis of arthritis in childhood. In: Southwood TR, Malleson PN (eds) Baillière's clinical paediatrics: arthritis in children and adolescents. Baillières Tindall, London; pp 665–695
22. Gedalia A, Press J 1991 Articular symptoms in hypermobile school children: a prospective study. Journal of Pediatrics 119:944–946
23. McConnell J 1986 Management of chondromalacia patellae – a long term solution. Australian Journal of Physiotherapy 32:215–225
24. Cicuttini F, Littlejohn GO 1989 Female adolescent presentations: the importance of chronic pain syndromes. Australian Paediatric Journal 25: 21–24

22 Acute management of complex regional pain syndrome type 1

Suellen Walker, Robert Eyres

Complex regional pain syndrome type 1 (CRPS-1), previously known as reflex sympathetic dystrophy, results in ongoing pain and disability following often minor injuries, and occurs in children[1-5] and adults. This condition is often not recognized in children, and thus patients may not receive optimal therapy.[1,6] The incidence of CRPS-1 is difficult to determine, owing to the lack of uniform terminology and diagnostic criteria in different medical disciplines and different countries. The term 'reflex sympathetic dystrophy' has lost clinical significance because no reflex is involved, the extent of sympathetic nervous system involvement in the generation of pain varies, and not all cases are associated with dystrophic changes. Complex regional pain syndrome type 2, previously referred to as 'causalgia', is a similar clinical syndrome but is associated with an identifiable nerve lesion.[7]

Sympathetically maintained pain (i.e. pain that is maintained by sympathetic efferent innervation or by circulating catecholamines) is frequently a component of complex regional pain syndromes. The relative contribution of sympathetically maintained pain to the overall pain state varies between individuals, or changes with time in a given patient. Thus, the degree of relief obtained with sympatholytic procedures may also vary.

CLINICAL FEATURES

Complex regional pain syndrome type 1 usually develops after an initiating noxious event; it is not limited to the distribution of a single peripheral nerve, and the pain is disproportionate to the severity of the inciting event. It is associated with some or all of the following: temperature changes, changes in skin blood flow and sudomotor activity (sweating), edema, bruising, allodynia (pain caused by a stimulus that does not normally provoke pain), and hyperalgesia (increased sensitivity to noxious stimuli).[5] The patient is typically protective of the painful region, and does not wish others to touch the involved limb. The pain may be described as burning, aching, throbbing, or lancinating.

Trophic changes are not invariably present, but in more chronic cases can manifest as muscle wasting, loss of hair, shiny parchment-like skin, and joint stiffness. In longstanding cases, decreased bone density may be seen on radiography, and limb shortening has been seen in a child with prolonged severe disease.[5]

The demography of CRPS-1 in pediatrics differs from that seen in adults.[1,2] In children and adolescents, CRPS-1 is more common in females (5:1), and in the author's experience the patient's personality is characterized by striving to achieve. The lower limbs are predominantly affected (8:1), with the right limb more often affected than the left (2:1). The initial injury incurred is often the result of sport, exercise, or dance. Early diagnosis is achieved by a high awareness of the condition in referring practitioners; it leads to earlier treatment, and gives the best chance of rapid recovery. In Wilder's series the average time to diagnosis was 1 year,[1] and patients required more prolonged treatment.

MANAGEMENT

Following referral, it is important to confirm the diagnosis of CRPS-1. The clinical symptoms and signs are the mainstay of diagnosis. Plain X-rays and bone scans should be considered, and comparison made with films of the unaffected limb. The main role of imaging is to exclude other conditions such as infection, stress fracture, osteoma, and rheumatoid conditions. Diffuse osteoporosis is seen in 20–30% of cases, and reflects disuse of affected limbs. Bone scans frequently show a diffuse increase in radionuclide tracer uptake in adults with CRPS-1. In children, decreased isotope uptake is more common. Accurate measurement of skin temperature or thermography may show an asymmetry between the affected and unaffected limb,[8] and can be useful in the assessment of therapy. Changes in skin potential recordings have also been used as an aid in diagnosis.[9]

An analgesic response to intravenous phentolamine is predictive of success with subsequent sympathetic blocks.[2,10,11] This technique has advantages as placebo-controlled infusions can be administered, it is relatively noninvasive and not painful, and therefore more readily accepted by children. Phentolamine is given in incremental doses, up to 0.5 mg/kg,[12] and blood pressure, heart rate, and visual analog pain score are monitored. In patients in whom the diagnosis is unclear, phentolamine may be used to determine if sympathetically maintained pain contributes to the pain syndrome, before proceeding to more invasive sympatholytic blocks.

In the Royal Children's Hospital, Melbourne, if symptoms and signs are highly suggestive of CRPS-1, the first step would be sympathetic nerve block with local anesthetic, as this is both a diagnostic and a therapeutic tool.

TREATMENT

Patients with CRPS-1 should be treated with a multidisciplinary approach. Persistent and aggressive therapy is essential because chronic cases may be more resistant to treatment. It is important to explain the nature of the disease and its expected course and management to the patients and their parents. Instant cures are uncommon, and thus all parties are liable to disappointment. The overall prognosis for CRPS-1 in children tends to be more favorable than in adults, with few progressing to atrophic changes, although relapses may occur.

The underlying or precipitating injury should be appropriately treated, to minimize nociceptive input from traumatized or inflamed tissue. The limb may have been immobilized as part of misguided therapy, or as a part of patient control of pain. The emphasis should be on mobilization and continuance of weight-bearing, before secondary changes of joint stiffness and atrophy of muscle and bone develop.

Subsequent treatment for CRPS-1 varies in different centers.[13] Physical therapy combined with a psychological program may be emphasized, with sympathetic blockade being reserved for patients who fail to progress. Alternatively, sympathetic blocks may be used early in the course of the disease, in conjunction with ongoing physiotherapy and mobilization. The role of sympathetic blocks is to relieve pain, allow physiotherapy to commence or continue, reverse physiological abnormalities of autonomic dysfunction, and restore function. Sympathetic blocks are generally felt to improve outcome and lead to more rapid resolution of symptoms, but adequate blinded trials have not been conducted.

Stellate ganglion blockade and lumbar sympathetic blockade with bupivacaine are the most common methods used to interrupt sympathetic innervation to the upper and lower limb respectively.[14] In older, cooperative adolescents, procedures may be performed with intravenous sedation, but general anesthesia is required in the majority of children. If the specific block is successful but the pain recurs in days or weeks, repeat blocks are indicated. Neurolytic blockade with phenol (3% or 6%) has been used in specific instances, but is rarely needed in pediatric practice. In patients with severe recurrent symptoms, a continuous epidural or sympathetic block (via a paravertebral catheter) may be required. Epidural clonidine has been used successfully in combination with dilute local anesthetic solution for refractory CRPS-1. Epidural infusions of 10–50 µg per hour of clonidine have been used to provide sustained analgesia in adults.[15] In children epidural clonidine is commenced at 0.2 µg/kg per hour, and the dose is increased if analgesia is inadequate and limiting side-effects of sedation and hypotension are absent.

Intravenous regional blocks are also used in children with CRPS-1.[13] Comparative trials between intravenous regional blocks and sympathetic ganglion blocks have not been performed, and preference for different techniques varies in different centers. Placement of intravenous catheters in edematous, hyperesthetic limbs may be difficult, and children with CRPS-1 may not tolerate an arterial tourniquet for 20 minutes without general anesthesia. Guanethidine (Ismelin) acts by blocking reuptake of norepinephrine (noradrenaline) and depleting peripheral adrenergic neuron stores. Following application of an arterial tourniquet, guanethidine 0.25 mg/kg in 10–20 ml is injected for the upper limb or 0.5 mg/kg in 20–30 ml for the lower limb. Pain on injection results from initial release of norepinephrine by guanethidine, but can be prevented by dilution in prilocaine 0.5% (maximum 3 mg/kg). Postural hypotension following tourniquet deflation is rare in children.[13] Intravenous regional blocks with bretylium, phenoxybenzamine, and ketorolac have also been used successfully.

A range of systemic drugs have been reported as beneficial in CRPS-1, but few are supported by large controlled trials, and the efficacy in children has not been adequately assessed. Phenoxybenzamine has been shown to be beneficial in some cases, but doses are limited by postural hypotension. Tricyclic antidepressants and anticonvulsants are frequently used in patients with neuropathic pain, and thus may be indicated in patients with associated nerve injuries. Anecdotal reports of phenytoin and gabapentin (an anticonvulsant with an improved side-effect profile)[16] describe beneficial effects in patients with CRPS-1. Nonsteroidal antiinflammatory drugs, calcitonin, corticosteroids, and nifedipine have been used in some centers.

Topical preparations of clonidine and guanethidine are undergoing trials in patients with CRPS-1, but may give only localized relief of symptoms in the area of application.

Transcutaneous electrical nerve stimulation (TENS), combined with physiotherapy, has been shown to benefit many children with CRPS-1.[1,17] As this therapy is noninvasive, more widespread use may be warranted, but controlled trials have not been performed.

Patients with longstanding CRPS-1 may require behavioral and cognitive therapies to break the pattern of disuse and fear of pain. Training in stress management and attention to family relationships may help eliminate 'secondary gain' such as avoiding school or family obligations, and promote coping behavior. A positive response to this therapy in patients with prolonged symptoms correlated with improved outcome.[1]

Increased recognition of CRPS in children and adolescents will result in earlier treatment, and minimize continuing pain and disability.

REFERENCES

1. Wilder RT, Berde CB, Wolohan M, Vieyra MA, Masek BJ, Micheli LJ 1992 Reflex sympathetic dystrophy in children. Journal of Bone and Joint Surgery 6:910–919.
2. Olsson GI, Arner S, Hirsch G 1990 Reflex sympathetic dystrophy in children. Advances in Pain Research and Therapy 15:323–331
3. Bernstein BH, Singsen BH, Kent JT et al 1978 Reflex neurovascular dystrophy in children. Journal of Pediatrics 93(2):211–215
4. Fermaglich DR 1977 Reflex sympathetic dystrophy in children. Pediatrics 60(6):881–883
5. Doolan LA, Brown TCK 1984 Reflex sympathetic dystrophy in a child. Anaesthesia and Intensive Care 12:70–72
6. Bickerstaff DR, Kanis JA 1994 Algodystrophy: an under-recognized complication of minor trauma. British Journal of Rheumatology 33:240–248
7. Stanton-Hicks M, Janig W, Hassenbusch S, Haddox JD, Boas R, Wilson P 1995 Reflex sympathetic dystrophy: changing concepts and taxonomy. Pain 63:127–133
8. Lightman HI, Pochaczevsky R, Prin H, Ilowite NT 1987 Thermography in childhood reflex sympathetic dystrophy. Journal of Pediatrics. 111(4):551–555
9. Cronin KD, Kirsner RLG 1979 Assessment of sympathectomy – the skin potential response. Anaesthesia and Intensive Care 7:353
10. Arner S 1991 Intravenous phentolamine test: diagnostic and prognostic use in reflex sympathetic dystrophy. Pain 46:17–22
11. Raja SN, Treede RD, Davis KD, Campbell JN 1991 Systemic alpha-adrenergic blockade with phentolamine: a diagnostic test for sympathetically maintained pain. Anesthesiology 74(4):691–698
12. Raja SN, Meleka SM, Turnquist JL, Campbell JN 1994 Monitoring adequacy of alpha-adrenoceptor blockade following systemic phentolamine administration. Thirteenth Annual Meeting American Pain Society Proceedings, A94721; p A-94.
13. Berde CJ, Olsson GI 1993 Neuropathic pain in children and adolescents. In: Schechter NL, Berde CB, Yaster M (eds) Pain in infants, children and adolescents, Williams & Wilkins, Baltimore, pp 473–494

14. Lofstrom JB, Cousins MJ 1988 Sympathetic neural blockade of upper and lower extremity. In: Cousins MJ, Bridenbaugh PO (eds) Neural blockade in clinical anesthesia and management of pain, 2nd edn. J B Lippincott, Philadelphia pp 461–502
15. Rauck RL, Eisenach JC, Jackson K, Young LD, Southern J 1993 Epidural clonidine treatment for refractory reflex sympathetic dystrophy. Anesthesiology 79:1163–1169
16. Mellick GA, Mellicy LB 1995 Gabapentin in the management of reflex sympathetic dystrophy. Journal of Pain Symptom Management 10:265–266
17. Kesler RW, Saulsbury FT, Miller LT, Rowlingson JC 1988 Reflex sympathetic dystrophy in children: treatment with transcutaneous electrical nerve stimulation. Pediatrics 82(5):728–732

FURTHER READING

Blumberg H, Janig W 1994 Clinical manifestations of reflex sympathetic dystrophy and sympathetically maintained pain. In: Wall PD, Melzack R (eds) Textbook of pain, 3rd edn. Churchill Livingstone, Edinburgh, pp 685–698
Bonica JJ 1990 Causalgia and other reflex sympathetic dystrophies. In: Bonica JJ (ed) The management of pain, 2nd edn. Lea & Febiger, Pennsylvania, pp 220–243
Janig W, Stanton-Hicks M (eds) 1996 Reflex sympathetic dystrophy: a reappraisal. Progress in pain research and management, vol 6. IASP, Seattle
Walker SM, Cousins MJ (in press) Complex regional pain syndromes: including 'reflex sympathetic dystrophy' and 'causalgia'. Anaesthesia and Intensive Care

23 Acute pain management services

Phil Gaukroger

Acute pain management services (APMS) have their origins in the introduction of chronic pain clinics in the 1960s. At that time it was common for
anesthesiologists with an interest in pain control to be referred chronic
pain patients, often with an expectation that some sort of nerve block
would be performed. Many clinicians involved in this area realized that
this approach to chronic pain was rarely effective and therefore introduced formal multidisciplinary chronic pain clinics. Interest in pain control expanded rapidly, with the number of pain clinics increasing, and the
appearance of professional bodies, journals, and conferences devoted
solely to pain control. The advances in diagnosis and treatment of illness
in the twentieth century had shifted the focus of medicine away from
symptom control. Chronic pain clinics and the renewed interest in pain
control set the scene for improving acute pain management.

In the 1970s and 1980s it was recognized that acute pain management,
especially postoperative pain management, was inadequate. During this
period, techniques that could improve the control of acute pain such as
nurse-controlled opioid infusions, patient-controlled analgesia (PCA), and
epidural infusions, were being developed, but required considerable
training of staff and specialist support. Ad hoc consultation about acute
pain problems was not an effective way of benefiting from these
advances. The problem of implementing improved acute pain management was commonly solved by introducing APMS to educate staff and
supervise new analgesia techniques. This is similar in concept to the introduction of other subspeciality branches of medicine or surgery.

The development of APMS for children followed in many major pediatric hospitals. These services have had to create protocols specifically for
children. For example, the fact that children are usually more upset than
adults by intramuscular injections means that this route is no longer routinely used in children but is reserved for specific indications. Nurse-controlled opioid infusions for younger children, PCA in older children, and
epidural infusions have assumed increasing importance. The next challenge is to bring the benefits of these advances to children in other hospitals. One of the roles of the APMS of a pediatric referral center is to assist
other institutions with their training and protocols for pain management
in children. The clinical support for consultation and resuscitation at these
centers may influence what techniques are used and whether they are
restricted to high dependency or intensive care units.

WHAT IS A PEDIATRIC ACUTE PAIN MANAGEMENT SERVICE?

Pediatric APMS vary immensely in the services they provide, their staffing and in their degree of funding. This variation is largely due to the differing needs of individual hospitals and their philosophy as to who should manage acute pain.

An adequately funded service in a large teaching hospital usually has both a full-time consultant and junior medical staff (most often anesthesiologists) and a full-time pain management nurse who are available 'in hours' to provide the service and attend patients who are being managed by the service. Most pediatric hospitals of this size will have 24 hour availability of anesthesia staff, usually senior trainees, who can respond to acute pain management problems after hours and liase with consultant staff if required, although some APMS provide a continuous direct consultant service.

The benefit of a formal APMS is that improved pain management techniques are quickly accepted because of the support provided to ward staff. Without the support of an APMS, changes in pain management are often perceived as burdensome and confusing. An APMS can provide rapid consultation, staff education, and clear protocols, and audit progress with both old and new techniques. These apparently simple tasks are difficult to achieve without having staff formally rostered to these duties. Providing staff and facilities for an APMS may seem a luxury to a hospital management inevitably restricted in funding, but the benefits in patient satisfaction and in outcome and staff morale are substantial. There are a number of ways in which these improvements may reduce costs.

When senior ward staff are trained and standard protocols for various pain management techniques are in place, the need for APMS consultations is reduced and the percentage of time spent in direct clinical care by the APMS may decrease. Accreditation of new staff in the management of various analgesic techniques, reaccreditation, audit, the introduction of new techniques, research, and (for a pediatric APMS) providing training in pediatric pain control for staff in other institutions are likely to consume a greater percentage of APMS time than patient contact.

Some centers have managed to improve pain management in children without a formal APMS. This usually involves one or several individuals (usually anesthesiologists often with ward nursing support) who educate, introduce protocols and consult on acute pain problems when available, although primary responsibility for the patient's analgesia remains with the ward staff. Leaving this responsibility with the ward nursing and medical staff has the benefit that they are able to coordinate all aspects of patient care including pain management. Another benefit of this system is low staff cost, but it is very dependent on the dedication of the individual or individuals coordinating the service and the cooperation of ward staff.

In centers with limited resources, this latter model can provide reasonable solutions to most acute pain management problems by the thoughtful use of simple analgesics (see Ch. 3), opioid infusions (in one simple form using only an intravenous giving set with a burette, see Ch. 5), and local anesthesia (see Chs 8, 9, and 20). The key to the success of the management lies more in the attitude, training, and support of staff (see Ch. 12) than in the availability of expensive equipment.

Most pediatric APMS lie between these two ends of the spectrum. However, the aims and essential features of these services are similar.

WHICH CHILDREN ARE MANAGED BY THE APMS?

The majority of adult APMS deal only with postoperative pain. In children's hospitals, APMS usually deal with a wider spectrum of acute pain including procedural pain, burns, oncology patients, and children requiring palliative care. These children usually benefit from having their pain management coordinated by an APMS and should be offered specialized techniques where appropriate.

In practice, the APMS usually has a direct clinical involvement with children receiving PCA, epidural analgesia, local anesthetic infusions (other than epidural), and other specialized techniques such as low-dose ketamine infusions. Children receiving an opioid infusion will often benefit from APMS consultation. Protocols for opioid infusions have become so well established in some centers that children having this treatment are not routinely reviewed by the APMS but managed by ward staff who request consultation as required. In many pediatric centers administration of nitrous oxide for control of acute procedural pain will be performed by the APMS. In other centers the APMS will be responsible for accreditation of staff in the use of this technique but will not necessarily administer the nitrous oxide in all cases.

Psychological techniques for pain management such as guided imagery (see Ch. 13) may be particularly useful for children with special fears or needs or requiring repeated interventions. An APMS may be able to train the child, the family, and the staff in these techniques. Initially, it may be helpful if a particular staff member with skills in this area attends each procedure, but the aim should be to train those involved to manage the techniques themselves.

Children with chronic noncancer pain are best managed by a multidisciplinary chronic pain service, not an APMS. The management of chronic pain has little in common with the management of acute pain. If there is no chronic pain clinic, the APMS will almost inevitably be asked to review patients with chronic pain. Members of the APMS will often realize that the child with chronic pain has many needs that are not being met, but the APMS does not have the resources to deal with these patients. In this situation, it may be useful to have a consultant with an understanding of chronic pain who can provide initial assessment and referral for these patients. Although this consultant may have duties with the APMS, it should be made clear that the management of these patients is not part of the APMS. Chronic pain patients will need a thorough assessment and, usually, referral to a number of disciplines, such as physiotherapy, psychology, neurology, social work, and others.

FUNCTIONS OF AN APMS

An APMS should:

1. Coordinate all techniques of acute pain management
2. Supervise specialized analgesic techniques
3. Teach and accredit medical and nursing staff
4. Institute and update protocols
5. Consult as required
6. Perform quality assurance activities
7. Conduct research
8. Manage and coordinate equipment and pharmaceuticals
9. Support all staff involved with acute pain management

Diplomacy and communication on a broad scale are important if an APMS is to succeed. The management of drug supplies and equipment may provide major administrative challenges for an APMS. The hospital pharmacy and biomedical engineering department (or equivalent) must be aided in providing what are often new devices and preparations to facilitate pain management. Budgetary policy may be crucial to the success of an APMS. It should be clarified whether funds for acute pain management will come from the APMS, the medical or surgical unit, or a central hospital budget. Most surgeons quickly recognize the benefits of improved pain management and are grateful for the support of an APMS. Occasionally disagreements will arise between the surgeon in charge of the patient and the APMS. Amicable reasoned compromise is in the best interests of all concerned, as it is likely to lead to further consultation with the APMS rather than alienation. These are just a few examples that emphasize the fact that the success of an APMS depends not only on the care of the patient but also on the care with which the APMS manages a wide range of staff in the hospital.

CONCLUSION

With the development of acute pain services for children, a rapid improvement in the management of pediatric pain has been evident. Acute pain management services are becoming an essential part of care, rather than a luxury, in pediatric hospitals.

Appendices

The following pages contain examples of forms that relate to acute pain management based on those used at the Royal Children's Hospital, Melbourne, Australia.

1. Opioid prescription form, 50 ml dilution (Appendix I)

2. Opioid prescription form, 500 ml dilution (Appendix I)

3. PCA prescription form (Appendix II)

4. PCA protocol (Appendix II)

5. Epidural prescription form (Appendix III)

6. Epidural protocol (Appendix III)

7. Pain management observation form (Appendix IV)

8. PCA patient and parent information form (Appendix V)

9. Epidural patient and parent information form (Appendix V)

These forms have been designed taking into account the particular circumstances of the Royal Children's Hospital. Other hospitals with different expertise, staff training, resuscitation support or availability of consultant advice will need to modify these forms. They are published here as a guide to some of the areas that should be addressed when introducing these analgesia techniques.

On each ward there is also a Royal Children's Hospital Pediatric Nursing Handbook which acts as a resource for staff. For specialized analgesia techniques nursing staff must be accredited by completing a 'learning package', and passing a practical and theoretical assessment.

APPENDIX I: OPIOID PRESCRIPTION FORMS

Opioid prescription form, 50 ml

ROYAL CHILDREN'S HOSPITAL, MELBOURNE

OPIOID INFUSION INSTRUCTIONS   AFFIX PATIENT IDENTIFICATION LABEL

Fifty (50) ml dilution

Weight.....................

GUIDELINES   TICK ☐   IF PRESCRIPTION DIFFERS FROM GUIDELINES

MORPHINE   Add **0.5 mg/kg** to **50 ml**
Infuse at **0–4 ml/h** (equivalent to 0–40 µg/kg·h)
Recommended initial bolus: 5 ml of infusion (50 µg/kg)
Recommended bolus for pain or painful procedures: 1–2 ml of infusion (10–20 µg/kg). Minimum 5–10 minutes between boluses

PETHIDINE   Add **5.0 mg/kg** to **50 ml**
Infuse at **0–4 ml/h** (equivalent to 0–0.4 mg/kg·h)
Recommended initial bolus: 5 ml of infusion (0.5 mg/kg)
Recommended bolus for pain or painful procedures: 1–2 ml of infusion (0.1–0.2 mg/kg). Minimum 5–10 minutes between boluses

MEDICAL INSTRUCTIONS

1. Add ....**mg** of .... to **50 ml** of ....

2. Infusion range: .... to .... **ml/h** as required for analgesia

3. Administer initial bolus .... **ml** of infusion

4. Administer .... ml bolus of infusion p.r.n. for pain or painful procedures, at intervals of no less than .... minutes

5. Notify doctor if respirations less than .... per minute or systolic blood pressure less than .... mmHg

6. Page APMS or on-duty anesthetic registrar for consultation

   IF EXCESSIVE OPIOID EFFECT SUSPECTED
   (slow or shallow respirations or hypotension or excess sedation)

1. Resuscitate as required ("ABC": Airway, Breathing, Circulation)
2. Call resuscitation team for assistance if required. Page APMS or on-duty anesthetic registrar for consultation
3. Administer oxygen. Monitor: SaO_2, BP, HR, RR, conscious state
4. Stop or decrease the opioid infusion
5. If instructed: Administer **NALOXONE** .... **IV** (2 to 100 µg/kg)
                  or NALOXONE .... **IM** (10 to 100 µg/kg)

Doctor's signature .... Date .... Printed name ....

INFUSION RECORD

INFUSION PREPARATION	Time & Date	Registered Nurses' Signatures
Syringe 1	....	....
Syringe 2	....	....
Syringe 3	....	....
Syringe 4	....	....
Syringe 5	....	....
Syringe 6	....	....

INFUSION DISCARDED

Syringe No:_____	....	....
Syringe No:_____	....	....

INITIAL BOLUS GIVEN: ....

For full details of the Hospital policy concerning opioid infusions please see "Opioid Infusions" in the Royal Children's Hospital Paediatric Nursing Handbook.

Opioid prescription form, 500 ml

ROYAL CHILDREN'S HOSPITAL, MELBOURNE

OPIOID INFUSION INSTRUCTIONS   AFFIX PATIENT IDENTIFICATION LABEL

Five hundred (500) ml dilution

Weight.....................

GUIDELINES   TICK ☐ IF PRESCRIPTION DIFFERS FROM GUIDELINES

MORPHINE   Add **0.5 mg/kg** to **500 ml**
Infuse at **0–40 ml/h** (equivalent to 0–40 µg/kg·h)
Recommended initial bolus: 50 ml of infusion (50 µg/kg)
Recommended bolus for pain or painful procedures: 10–20 ml of infusion (10–20 µg/kg). Minimum 5–10 minutes between boluses

PETHIDINE   Add **5.0 mg/kg** to **500 ml**
Infuse at **0–40 ml/h** (equivalent to 0–0.4 mg/kg·h)
Recommended initial bolus: 50 ml of infusion (0.5 mg/kg)
Recommended bolus for pain or painful procedures: 10–20 ml of infusion (0.1–0.2 mg/kg). Minimum 5–10 minutes between boluses

MEDICAL INSTRUCTIONS

1. Add ....**mg** of .... to **500 ml** of ....

2. Infusion range: .... to .... **ml/h** as required for analgesia

3. Administer initial bolus .... **ml** of infusion

4. Administer .... ml bolus of infusion p.r.n. for pain or painful procedures, at intervals of no less than .... minutes

5. Notify doctor if respirations less than .... per minute or systolic blood pressure less than .... mmHg

6. Page APMS or on-duty anesthetic registrar for consultation

   IF EXCESSIVE OPIOID EFFECT SUSPECTED
   (slow or shallow respirations or hypotension or excess sedation)

1. Resuscitate as required ("ABC": Airway, Breathing, Circulation)
2. Call resuscitation team for assistance if required. Page APMS or on-duty anesthetic registrar for consultation
3. Administer oxygen. Monitor: SaO_2, BP, HR, RR, conscious state
4. Stop or decrease the opioid infusion
5. If instructed: Administer **NALOXONE** .... **IV** (2 to 100 µg/kg)
                              or NALOXONE .... **IM** (10 to 100 µg/kg)

Doctor's signature .... Date .... Printed name ....

INFUSION RECORD

INFUSION PREPARATION	Time & Date	Registered Nurses' Signatures
Bag 1	....	....
Bag 2	....	....
Bag 3	....	....
Bag 4	....	....
Bag 5	....	....
Bag 6	....	....

INFUSION DISCARDED

Bag No:_____	....	....
Bag No:_____	....	....

INITIAL BOLUS GIVEN: .... | ....
For full details of the Hospital policy concerning opioid infusions please see "Opioid Infusions" in the Royal Children's Hospital Paediatric Nursing Handbook.

APPENDIX II: PCA PRESCRIPTION FORM AND PROTOCOL

PCA prescription form

ROYAL CHILDREN'S HOSPITAL, MELBOURNE

ACUTE PAIN MANAGEMENT SERVICE

PATIENT-CONTROLLED ANALGESIA – PRESCRIBING INFORMATION SHEET

UNIT:....................

WEIGHT:........... kg   **BRADMA LABEL**

PROCEDURE:...

ANALGESIA IN THEATRE:...

....

PCA REGIMEN

- **0.5 mg/kg morphine or 5 mg/kg pethidine (meperidine)**
- **Diluted to a total volume of 50 ml with normal saline**

Note: Morphine is the preferred agent in most circumstances for children due to the concern of normeperidine toxicity which can result when meperidine is used.

PCA PROGRAM (Usual Protocol)

- Bolus dose: morphine 2 ml / 20 µg/kg
- Lockout interval: 5 minutes
- Background infusion: (optional) morphine 0.5 ml/h (5 µg/kg/h)
- Loading dose/programming of the PCA machine should only be operated by an anesthetist or the Acute Pain Management Service

P.C.A. SETTINGS

Add .... mg ☐ morphine ☐ pethidine (meperidine) and dilute to a total of 50 ml with

normal saline =..............mg/ml.

Date/Time	Bolus (mg/mls)	Dose Duration	Lockout (mins)	Concentration (mg/ml)	Background (ml/h)	Signature

Any problems contact:
Acute Pain Management Service: Pager XXXX
In charge anesthetist / after hours anesthetic registrar: Extension XXXX

PCA protocol

ROYAL CHILDREN'S HOSPITAL – ACUTE PAIN MANAGEMENT SERVICE

PATIENT-CONTROLLED ANALGESIA – PROTOCOL

Patient-controlled analgesia (PCA) is a technique for managing *acute* pain which utilizes a programmable syringe pump to allow patients to *self-administer* their own intravenous opioid medication.

ADVANTAGES

- Less complications when opioids are administered in this way
- Excellent analgesia for the majority of patients
- High patient satisfaction
- Increased nursing satisfaction

Further information can be obtained from the Staff Information Sheet.

INDICATIONS

Management of all forms of acute and acute-on-chronic pain, e.g. surgically related, postoperative burns, oncology, frequent painful dressing changes

CONTRAINDICATIONS

- Inability to understand the concept of pressing a button when you need pain relief (e.g. pre-school children)
- Head injury
- Severe intercurrent illness, such as asthma, cardiac disease
- Previous severe adverse reactions from opioid drugs

N.B. All these contraindications are relative, and therefore should be discussed with the department of anesthesia.

HOW TO ARRANGE PCA

- PCA is a specialized technique and must be commenced and supervised by the Acute Pain Management Service and anesthesia staff
- An accredited Registered Nurse (RN) is one who has successfully completed the PCA Learning Package. Only accredited registered nursing staff should manage a patient on PCA therapy
- PCA units are available from the Central Equipment Pool, located in the Recovery Room
- Two *inoperable* PCA pumps and hand sets are located in unit 3 West for educational purposes
- Contact unit 3 West to arrange to utilize a pump for a patient education session

PRESCRIPTION OF PCA

The prescription of PCA is only performed by anesthetic staff
ONLY anesthetists, recovery nurses or the Acute Pain Management service members can program the PCA
If appropriate an accredited registered nurse may be instructed by the Acute Pain Management Service or anesthetist to change the program parameters of the PCA machine.

PCA ORDERS ARE WRITTEN:

- On the PCA prescribing information sheet
- On the medication sheet where indicated by the appropriate drug order sticker
- Orders to be reviewed every 24 hours by the Acute Pain Management Service

SYRINGE CHANGES:

- Syringes should be changed every 24 hours
- A countersigned additive label should be attached

- All syringe changes should be signed for by the registered nurses on the medication chart
- Syringe changes are performed by accredited nursing staff. If any problems are encountered, then the instruction manual should be consulted or the Acute Pain Management Service or anesthetist on call notified

REGIMEN

0.5 mg/kg morphine

or   } are diluted up to a total volume of 50 ml with normal saline

5 mg/kg pethidine (meperidine)

Morphine is the preferred agent in most circumstances due to the concern of normeperidine toxicity which can result when pethidine (meperidine) is used.

The usual settings the machine is programmed to by the anesthetist are:
- Bolus dose size = 2 ml = 20 µg/kg **morphine**
- Lockout interval = 5 minutes
- Background infusion (optional) of 0.5 ml/h (5 µg/kg·h) **morphine**

These settings are outlined on the PCA prescribing information sheet.
Any requests for change of settings are referred to the Acute Pain Management Service or department of anesthesia.

ANTIREFLUX VALVE

- If a gravity-fed intravenous line or 'Y' line is being used in conjunction with PCA therapy an antireflux valve is required
- An antireflux valve is necessary to prevent accumulation of the opioid in the line should the intravenous cannula become blocked or kinked

FOLLOW-UP

- Patient will be reviewed daily by the Acute Pain Management Service or anesthetic department
- Cessation of PCA therapy must be done in consultation with the APMS. This may involve initially ceasing the background infusion where applicable, then after review the demand mode, or by ceasing the complete infusion
- An oral analgesic should be prescribed
- PCA is available to all appropriate patients in both surgical and medical units which have PCA accredited registered nurses available

OBSERVATIONS

- **RESPIRATORY RATE, PULSE RATE – HOURLY UNTIL INFUSION CEASED**
- Blood pressure readings fourth hourly unless otherwise indicated
- Syringe level **MUST** be recorded hourly on the fluid balance chart
- Patient's pain, sedation, vomiting score, number of demands, deliveries and dose (mg/h) should be documented hourly
- All data should be recorded on the PCA observation chart

The need for less frequent observations on patients with longer-term PCA should be discussed with the Acute Pain Management Service.

PCA POSITION

The PCA pump must be positioned at or below the patient's chest level, so if the syringe is not airtight, siphoning will not occur.

COMPLICATIONS

If respiratory rate < 10/min, or respiratory depression or oversedation is suspected:

- Stop PCA therapy
- Administer oxygen therapy
- Maintain i.v. access

- Ensure suction equipment is available
- Resuscitate
- Ventilate
- Prepare naloxone (Narcan) 0.01 mg/kg i.v. to be administered immediately
- Notify anesthetist on call if the patient unrousable or apneic

PORTABLE PCA

Older children on day 2 or 3 of PCA therapy may be suitable for non-electronic PCA (patient controlled injector).

Principles are the same as above, but REGIMEN is:
1 mg/kg in 25 ml saline (40 μg/ml)
Bolus size: 0.5 ml
Lockout: 5-minutes
No background

SPECIAL NOTE

This protocol was devised considering the skills, training and availability of nursing and medical staff at the RCH. The protocol may be unsuitable in other institutions.

APPENDIX III: EPIDURAL PRESCRIPTION FORM AND PROTOCOL

Epidural prescription form

ROYAL CHILDREN'S HOSPITAL

ACUTE PAIN MANAGEMENT SERVICE – EPIDURAL INFUSION CHART

PATIENT DATA

Weight:....................kg

Operation: . . . .

Surgeon: . . . .   **BRADMA LABEL**

Anesthetist: . . . .

Date/Time of operation: . . . .

EPIDURAL TECHNIQUE	**EPIDURAL FORMULATION**

Level: . . . .   Bupivacaine. . . . .% in . . . . . . ml

Needle gauge: . . . .   Fentanyl. . . . . .μg/ml

Catheter position at skin . . . . .cm   Commencement Rate:. . . . . .ml/h

Problems: At insertion: . . . .

Intraoperative: . . . .

OBSERVATIONS

- **Commencement of Infusion:**
  Hourly PR/RR/BP for 4 hours

- **Routine:**
  Once patient stable and comfortable – hourly PR/RR, 4-hourly BP
  Note: A patient at risk of hypotension may require hourly BP at the discretion of the anesthetist

- **Post bolus:**
  Five minutely PR/RR/BP for 20 minutes then PR/RR/BP 1 hour post bolus
  If patient stable and comfortable – then routine observations

- If the block needs to be reestablished with a bolus of 0.25% or 0.5% bupivacaine, a nonstandard concentration, drug or volume, this must be performed by an anesthetist
  The anesthetist **MUST** remain in unit for 20 minutes following this bolus

- **Increase of Rate:**
  Commencement observations then routine observations

NOTIFIABLE – IMMEDIATELY CONTACT ANESTHETIC DEPARTMENT

BP(Systolic)	>	<		– inadequate analgesia
HR	>	<	**AND/OR**	– decreased conscious state
RR	>	<		– numbness/tingling in fingers, arms
				– decreased oxygen saturation
				– arrhythmias

MANAGEMENT OF INFUSION (Change of flask)

Bupivacaine 0.125% with or without fentanyl may be administered after consultation with APMS or Anesthetist on call.
BOLUS (accredited registered nurses only)

If bolus dose required:

1. Notify APMS or anesthetist oncall
2. Bupivacaine (0.125%) .... ml stat. via activation of quick feed button on syringe infusion pump
3. Notify above persons if analgesia ineffective 15 minutes after bolus
4. Please note on back of this chart administration of bolus and effect

Anesthetist's signature .... Date......./......../........

NO OTHER OPIOID OR SEDATIVE AGENTS to be given to the patient while epidural infusion in progress without prior
consultation with an anesthetist.

CONTACT IF PROBLEMS

- Acute Pain Management Service: Pager XXXX
- In-charge anesthetist: Extension XXXX
- After 1800 hours/weekends – On-duty anesthetic registrar: Extension XXXX

Note: Any change in infusion solution bolus administration, or rate must be detailed below.

Date/Time	Solution % +/– Fentanyl	Infusion rate	Bolus % ml administered	Effect of bolus Comments	RN Sign	Anaes. Sign

EPIDURAL CATHETER REMOVAL DETAILS

Date/Time:

Catheter tip intact: YES / NO

Epidural site: ....
....

Signature: ....

**IF CATHETER TIP NOT INTACT PLEASE KEEP THE CATHETER AND INFORM THE ANESTHETIC DEPARTMENT
IMMEDIATELY**

NOTE: PLEASE RETURN THIS COMPLETED CHART TO ANESTHETIC DEPARTMENT

Epidural protocol

ROYAL CHILDREN'S HOSPITAL

ACUTE PAIN MANAGEMENT SERVICE – EPIDURAL INFUSION PROTOCOL

- Patient suitability for a continuous epidural infusion is to be determined by anesthetist. The anesthetist should discuss the intention to use an epidural infusion with the Unit Nursing Staff prior to commencement
- The anesthetist will discuss all aspects of the epidural infusion with the parents and patient, a separate consent form is not required. An information sheet for parents and patient (if applicable) is available
- Epidural catheters are inserted by the anesthetist in theater. The infusion will be commenced during anesthesia or in the recovery room after surgery
- Infusions will all be run via a syringe pump. These pumps are available from a central equipment pool located in the recovery room
- A continuous epidural infusion can be implemented on the unit provided sufficient epidural accredited nursing staff are available
- Bupivacaine 0.125% (Marcain) is usually the solution prescribed. Fentanyl 2 μg/ml may be added, often for the first 24 hour period of the infusion. On review by APMS or the anesthetist, the fentanyl maybe continued or ceased
- Prepared flasks of 0.125% bupivacaine of 100 and 200 ml are used. The standard solutions of local anesthetic with or without fentanyl are available through the Hospital Pharmacy Department

These flasks should be kept on Unit imprest and if containing fentanyl in the Dangerous Drug cupboard

- If required after pharmacy hours, nonstandard epidural infusion solutions can be prepared by the anesthetist on duty. Nursing staff should give advance notification if they require the anesthetist to prepare the prescribed solution

---

OBSERVATIONS

- **Commencement of Infusion:**
  hourly PR/RR/BP for 4 hours

- **Routine:**
  once patient stable and comfortable – hourly PR/RR, 4-hourly BP
  Note: A patient at risk of hypotension may require hourly BP at the discretion of the anesthetist.

- **Post Bolus:**
  5-minutely PR/RR/BP for 20 minutes then PR/RR/BP 1 hour post bolus
  If patient stable and comfortable – then routine observations
- If the block needs to be reestablished with a bolus of 0.25% or 0.5% bupivacaine, a nonstandard concentration, drug or volume, this must be performed by an anesthetist
  The anesthetist **MUST** remain in unit for 20 minutes following this bolus

- **Increase of Rate:**
  commencement observations then routine observations

SITE

- The epidural site should be observed at least once a shift
- Observe the epidural dressing and the epidural insertion site for any redness, discharge, lump or leakage of fluid
- Any abnormality should be reported to the Acute Pain Management Service or an anesthetist
- If a minimal leakage of epidural solution is present and the patient is comfortable suggesting the epidural is providing analgesia, the area can be redressed. If a large leak is present **after consultation** with the APMS the infusion may be ceased and the epidural catheter removed
- The catheter position should also be observed to ensure it is in the correct position. This is done by checking the catheter's markings and referring to the epidural prescribing information sheet

---

DERMATOMAL LEVEL

- Where appropriate a dermatomal level should be assessed by light touch or cold sensation to establish the level at which the sensation changes
- The solution infused is usually 0.125% bupivacaine and due to its low concentration it maybe difficult to ascertain the loss of dermatomal sensation

PAIN ASSESSMENT

- The patient must be assessed for any pain. Pain rating scores using developmentally appropriate scales must be taken hourly (except if the patient is asleep) until 4 hours after the infusion is ceased
- Thereafter provided the patient is comfortable, 4-hourly pain ratings can be taken
- These ratings must be recorded on the epidural observation chart

RECORDING THE EPIDURAL INFUSION

- For legal prescribing purposes the concentration of bupivacaine and fentanyl used in the infusion should be written and signed for by the anesthetist on the *patient's medication chart*
- Adhesive-backed labels are provided which alert medical and nursing staff to avoid the concurrent use of other opioids/sedative agents. These labels are attached to the epidural prescribing chart
- Epidural infusion prescribing charts are available in the recovery room. The chart is to be filled out by the anesthetist, outlining details about the solution prescribed, catheter, infusion rate and observation parameters
- Any change in epidural infusion rate, administration of a bolus, or change of epidural infusion solution should be recorded on this chart
- Contents of syringe needs to be recorded on the syringe via an additive label
- When an epidural flask is replaced, the RN must sign in the appropriate place on the patient's medication chart, also recording the volume of the flask (pharmacy requirement)
- The syringe infusion level should be checked by the nursing staff every hour, and documented on the fluid balance chart

REVIEW

- The Acute Pain Management Service or the in-charge anesthetist will review all problems with the infusions, including inadequacy of analgesia and problems with the syringe pumps
- The Acute Pain Management Service can be contacted each weekday between 0800 and 1800 hours: Pager XXXX
- If required the in-charge consultant anesthetist can be contacted: Extension XXXX
- If required after hours and on weekends the duty anesthetic registrar can be contacted: Extension XXXX

BOLUS ADMINISTRATION

- If analgesia is inadequate a bolus of local anesthetic may be given and the infusion rate may be changed after consultation with the anesthetic department
- Where possible this bolus dose should be administered by an anesthetist. If the anesthetist is occupied in the operating room and unable to attend immediately, a phone order to administer a prescribed bolus from the syringe pump may be given to the Unit nurse
- A nurse accredited in epidural infusion management may give a bolus of 0.125% bupivacaine with or without fentanyl, as per written order or phone order (according to patient's weight and size), of the solution in the syringe. It may **ONLY** be given by activating the quick feed mechanism on the pump, not by manually pushing the syringe

CESSATION

- The cessation of the epidural infusion therapy should be done in consultation with the APMS
- Oral analgesia should be given 1 hour after cessation of the infusion
- Educate the parents and where applicable the child about the possibility of the child being a little unsettled as the anesthetic wears off, as they no longer feel any loss of sensation (approximately 2 hours after cessation). The child should not experience any acute episodes of pain; if they do the APMS should be notified.

REMOVAL

- Remove the tape from the child's back and shoulder
- Position the child either laterally or bending forward, which opens the vertebral bodies, making removal easier
- Wearing sterile gloves, gently withdraw the catheter

- Check catheter tip and epidural site
- Place adhesive plaster over the area
- Complete the documentation

CONCURRENT DRUGS

- If epidural opioids are used, NO ORAL / PR / INTRAVENOUS OR INTRAMUSCULAR opioids or sedatives agents should be given without prior consultation with an anesthetist
- Pain at sites other than the surgical wound, i.e. N/G tubes, IV lines may require supplementary analgesic cover with oral or rectal paracetamol (acetominophen)

NURSING MANAGEMENT

- The duration of the epidural infusion will depend on the patient's analgesic requirements, but the infusion should rarely be required for longer than 72 hours
- Intravenous access is mandatory in any patient with an epidural catheter in situ, to administer intravenous fluids if the patient is hypotensive or requires naxolone to be administered.
  Access is to remain in place till the local anesthetic agent and/or opioid agent has worn off (usually 2–4 hours) following cessation of the infusion
- The epidural giving set should **NOT** have a drug port, thus preventing accidental drug administration
- At completion of the infusion an anesthetist or accredited registered nurse will remove the epidural catheter. The nurse or anesthetist who removes the epidural catheter is required to check the catheter tip to ensure it is intact, and check the epidural insertion site for any abnormalities. The person who removes the catheter is required to complete the necessary documentation which is located on the back of the epidural prescribing information chart. The completed prescribing chart is then sent to the Acute Pain Management Service via the anesthetic department
- In this protocol an 'Accredited Registered Nurse' refers to a nurse who has satisfactorily completed the Epidural Learning Package at RCH and whose accreditation is current

NOTE: This protocol was devised considering the skills, training and availability of nursing and medical staff at the RCH The protocol may be unsuitable for use in other institutions.

APPENDIX IV: PAIN MANAGEMENT OBSERVATION FORM

RCH ACUTE PAIN MANAGEMENT SERVICE
PCA / EPIDURAL / OPIOID INFUSION
OBSERVATION & PAIN RATING CHART   **BRADMA LABEL**

Date Commenced:...../....../......

PLEASE RETURN THIS FORM TO THE ANESTHETIC DEPARTMENT AT THE CONCLUSION OF INFUSION

Time	Pulse	Resp	B.P.	P. Pain Score	Par. Pain Score	Sed'n Score	Vomit Score	Comments	Total Tries		Hourly Tries		Total (mg) Dosage
									Good	Bad	Good	Bad	
1:00													
2:00													
3:00													
4:00													
5:00													
6:00													
7:00													
8:00													
9:00													
10:00													
11:00													
12:00													
13:00													
14:00													
15:00													
16:00													
17:00													
18:00													
19:00													
20:00													
21:00													
22:00													
23:00													
24:00													

SEDATION
SCORE
1=Awake
2=Drowsy
3=Asleep

VOMITING
SCORE
0=Nil
1=Nausea
2=Vomiting in Last Hour

OBSERVATIONS

As per relevant protocol

PAIN RATING SCORE 1/24 until infusion ceased.

Note: Indicate which pain scale in use by ticking relevant box.

☐	VISUAL ANALOG SCALE (0–10)
☐	PAIN DESCRIPTION 0=no pain, 1-mild pain, 2=moderate pain, 3=severe pain
☐	WONG-BAKER FACES (0–5)

APPENDIX V: PATIENT AND PARENT INFORMATION FORMS

PCA patient and parent information form

ROYAL CHILDREN'S HOSPITAL – ACUTE PAIN MANAGEMENT SERVICE

PATIENT CONTROLLED ANALGESIA

PATIENT / PARENT INFORMATION SHEET

When PCA therapy is discussed with the patient and their family, often many questions arise. This information sheet will help answer the most common questions. If you have any other questions, please ask the doctors or nurses.

1. **What is PCA?**
   Patient-controlled analgesia (PCA) is a technique which enables the patient to administer their own analgesia (pain relief medicine) when they require it. The technique is devised so that it is safe with standard supervision by the ward staff.

2. **Why does the patient control how much pain relief medicine they need?**
   The patient is often the best judge of how much pain they have, when they have pain, and how much pain relief medicine (analgesia) they require to decrease their pain to a level which they can tolerate. The PCA should allow the patient to deep breathe, cough, move around in bed, and participate in normal activities after surgery.

3. **What is a PCA Machine?**
   You may have already been shown the PCA machine. This machine is programmed to deliver a specially calculated dose of analgesia (usually morphine) when the button is pressed and not deliver any more until enough time has passed for that dose to work (usually about 5 minutes). Pushing the button during that time will not deliver any drug.

4. **Why do we measure/rate your pain and how?**
   When you are receiving treatment to relieve pain it is important for the doctor and nurses to know whether and how well the treatment is working.
   To help the doctor and nurses they will ask you to use a pain rating scale on which you either use a certain word to describe your pain at that time i.e. nil, mild, moderate, severe, or 'rate' your pain out of 10, 0 meaning no pain, 10 meaning the worst possible pain you have ever experienced.
   Some children prefer to point to one of a series of specially drawn faces to show how much pain they have. You and the nurses can discuss which type of scale you would like to use.

5. **When should I push the button?**
   If your pain is at a level which is causing you to feel uncomfortable then you should push the button so a dose of pain relief medicine can be administered.

6. **Will all the pain go away?**
   It is important that you understand that the pain you are experiencing will probably not completely go away using the PCA machine. The aim is to decrease the pain to a level which you can tolerate and be able to function as near to normal as possible.

7. **What other things can I do to help me manage my pain?**
   For mild pain you should try to do relaxation exercises such as deep breathing, imagining nice things you like to do, listen to music, or try some distraction activities such as watching television, playing video games or reading. Such things can calm you down, relax your muscles which can help you cope more effectively with your pain.
   If you don't know what to do, ask the nurse for suggestions.

8. **Can I give myself too much pain relief medicine?**
   No, there are several reasons for this. If you keep pushing the button when you don't have any pain, the medicine would make you fall asleep, thus you wouldn't be able to continue to press the button.
   The machine is also programmed so it will not give a dose of analgesia every time you push the button. Several minutes have to elapse between each dose to ensure that the medicine has had time to work effectively. This is called the 'lock-out time'.

9. **Who may press the button?**
   ONLY the patient may press the button when they have too much pain, as only they know how much pain they have. If anyone else pushes the button, it could result in serious complications for the patient, and the PCA therapy may have to be discontinued.
   If, as a parent, you feel your child is using the PCA inappropriately, e.g. lying in pain because they feel sick when they push the button, please tell the doctor or nurses, so they can help.

10. **What happens if I feel sick or itchy?**
    Sometimes the medicine we use to help control your pain can make you feel sick or itchy. Let the nurses know and they will be able to help you.

11. **Why do nurses ask me so many questions about my pain each hour?**
    The nurses will observe you frequently to ensure everything is satisfactory, and that you are managing your pain with your PCA therapy.

12. **How long will I have the machine for?**
    This depends on your individual requirements and the type of operation you have.
    Most patients require PCA for 2–3 days.

13. **What is the Pain Management Service?**
    This is a team of people (doctors and nurses) who review patients on PCA therapy each day. If you have any questions or concerns about PCA, please ask them.

Epidural patient and parent information form

ROYAL CHILDREN'S HOSPITAL – ACUTE PAIN MANAGEMENT SERVICE

POSTOPERATIVE EPIDURAL ANALGESIA

PARENT & PATIENT INFORMATION SHEET

This overview of epidural analgesia has been designed to answer questions often raised by parents and patients. If you have further queries, please ask the anesthetist or nursing staff.

1. **What is epidural analgesia?**
   For many years epidural analgesia has been used during childbirth. At the Royal Children's Hospital, epidural infusions have been used to provide postoperative pain relief (analgesia). With the development of new equipment, epidural infusions can be safely used in babies, infants and children.
   A small plastic catheter is inserted into the epidural space in the back under general anesthesia. Through this catheter, local anesthetic drugs and other pain-relieving drugs (similar to morphine) can be continuously administered via a special pump.

2. **Where is the epidural space?**
   The epidural space is located around and below the spinal cord from the base of the skull to the lower back area. This space contains fat, blood vessels and nerves. It is separated from the spinal cord and fluid by a membrane called the dura. Nerves from the spinal cord pass through this space to reach other areas of the body. Placing local anesthetic and pain-relieving drugs into this area will temporarily numb these nerves and thereby prevent the sensation of pain.

3. **What drugs are used and why?**
   By using a low dose of local anesthetic drug only the nerves conducting pain sensation will be blocked. Other nerves for movement are blocked to a much lesser degree and therefore patients are usually able to move about in bed. This is called selective sensory blockade.
   A pain-relieving drug like morphine (usually fentanyl) is often added to the local anesthetic drug, as they work more effectively together in some situations.

4. **What types of operations is epidural analgesia used for?**
   Epidurals have been successfully used for major surgery on the chest, abdomen, and legs. Not all operations or patients are suitable for this type of pain relief. The anesthetist can advise you about what is suitable for you.

5. **How long will the epidural be needed?**
   The infusions are started in the operating room by the anesthetist and usually continue in the ward for several days. Progress will be reviewed closely by the Acute Pain Management Service and anesthetists in conjunction with the nursing staff.

6. **Why are epidurals used?**
   Continuous epidural infusions offer a number of advantages. Excellent pain relief can be provided without the problems seen with opioid (i.e. morphine) intravenous infusions. Patients are less sedated, have less vomiting and recover bowel function more quickly than with other pain relieving methods and may have a shorter stay in hospital.

7. **What complications may occur?**
   This technique can have complications. The risks are very low, although the incidence of specific risks is difficult to quantitate. Risks include:

   1. Low blood pressure: this is unlikely with the low concentration of anesthetic drugs and is uncommon in children. It is usually treated with intravenous fluids.
   2. Back discomfort: some discomfort may be experienced at the site where the catheter enters the back. This is usually temporary, like a 'bruise' from the injection.
   3. Headache can occur if some fluid around the spinal cord leaks out through the dura. This is uncommon, usually settles, and can be effectively treated if necessary.
   4. Infection: very rare. More likely if the patient has poor immune function or existing infection.
   5. Bleeding: very rare. Any patient with a known bleeding disorder is excluded from having an epidural.
   6. Nerve damage: extremely rare. An area of weakness or numbness may occur and is usually transient. More serious nerve damage is even less likely.

8. **Possible infusion problems**
   Problems on the ward with these infusions are generally due to:

   1. Catheter problems: i.e. it blocks or moves from its correct position. Blockage may be overcome by pulling the catheter back slightly. If the problem remains the catheter may need to be removed completely. Catheters occasionally leak, also, and this is usually of no consequence.

2. Incomplete pain relief: the anesthetist will review and may alter the drug concentration, the rate of infusion or add additional drugs. If the pain relief remains inadequate the epidural will be ceased and other pain relief provided. There are many ways of assessing if the epidural is working and the patient is comfortable, such as testing where they are numb and where they have normal sensation. Pain rating scales are also used as a means for the child to communicate their intensity and location of pain to the doctors and nurses.

9. **Frequent observations**
    Temperature, pulse rate, respiratory rate and blood pressure will be taken. This is done to ensure the child's epidural is working effectively.

10. **How is the catheter removed?**
    At the completion of the infusion, the catheter is simply slipped out of the back. This is painless and requires no anesthetic.

Index